Take Me to Paris, Johnny

John Foster was born in Melbourne in 1944. After completing an Arts degree at Melbourne University, he studied extensively in Germany and the UK. He returned to Melbourne in 1971 when he took up a position in the Department of History at Melbourne University. He is also the author of *Community of Fate: Memoirs of German Jews in Melbourne* and *Victorian Picturesque: The Colonial Gardens of William Sangster*. John Foster died in 1994.

Praise for *Take Me to Paris, Johnny*

'Not only some kind of literary masterpiece, but a work of such grace and gravity, filled with such sparkle as well as sorrow, that it is, to my knowledge, unparalleled in Australian letters.'

– Peter Craven

'As it moves across continents, the story of a love affair between an Australian academic and a Cuban dancer reminds us of the complexity of relationships in a world of growing interconnections, and of the simultaneous strength and fragility of love.'

– Dennis Altman, author of *Defying Gravity* and *Global Sex*

'A story that resonates ... With its brilliantly accomplished use of language, *Take Me to Paris, Johnny* shows why love in one of its myriad forms can rescue lives from futility.'

– Robert Dessaix, author of *Night Letters*

Take Me to Paris, Johnny

JOHN FOSTER

Published by Black Inc.
An imprint of Schwartz Publishing
Level 5, 289 Flinders Lane
Melbourne Victoria 3000 Australia
email: enquiries@blackincbooks.com
www.blackincbooks.com

Text set in Granjon by Thomas Deverall

Printed in Australia by Griffin Press

National Library of Australia Cataloguing-in-Publication entry

Foster, J. H. (John Harvey), 1944-1994.
Take me to Paris, Johnny.

Rev. ed.
ISBN 1 86395 101 6.

1. Foster, J. H. (John Harvey), 1944-1994. 2. Céspedes,
Juan Gualberto, 1953-1987. 3. Gay male couples - Biography.
4. AIDS (Disease) - Patients - Biography. I. Title.

362.196979200922

CONTENTS

Acknowledgements

My affectionate thanks to the friends who, in various ways, helped me complete this memoir: Louise Adler, Ann Brady, Juliet Flesch, Rosemary Hogan, Hiram Pulzan, John Rickard, Elizabeth Ward and Heidi Zogbāum.

FOREWORD

Every so often a book comes along that reverses every expec-
tation you have about its subject matter and its presumed
style and leaves you feeling humble as well as grateful.
Take Me to Paris, Johnny is just such a book. It was no doubt
wrong, because unthinking, to imagine that a book about a
lover, dead of AIDS, was bound to be both sentimental and
depressing, but there was no particular reason to imagine
that the historian John Foster would produce a homage to
his partner Juan Céspedes which is not only some kind of
literary masterpiece but a work of such grace and gravity,
filled with such sparkle as well as sorrow, that it is, to my
knowledge, unparalleled in Australian letters.

It begins with the narrator journeying to Cuba, the
homeland of his lover, now more than a year dead, and the
prose warns us that we are in the presence of a writer it
would be insulting to describe as a stylist because he is so
much more.

From Santiago de Cuba the road ran east through the
central valley of the province. The country was exactly
as I wanted it to be – red earth, banana plantations and

hills that were crowned with a darker canopy of royal palms. Across the rising terrain to the north lay the Sierra del Cristal where Fidel Castro's brother had opened up the second front of the Revolution. Ahead, beyond the hills, were the Atlantic beaches of Baracoa where Columbus once claimed the island for the Spanish Crown. In the cathedral of the town – so they say – is preserved the cross that he planted in the sand. Later, when it was encased in precious metals and exposed to the veneration of the faithful, it brought them good fortune. Or, to put the matter more circumspectly, it rendered their fortunes less evil than they might otherwise have been. This was no mean blessing, for it is difficult to conceive how they could have borne more suffering then they did endure: slavery, revolt and civil war. Since the triumph of the Revolution, according to my driver, the efficacy of the cross had declined. By what measure this diminished power was established he did not say, and I reflected privately that in matters of unbelief a certain scepticism was required.

He has come to see the mother of Juan, a woman whose letters bespeak a passionate if stony dignity. 'I must tell you that on Mother's Day I received no letter from you which gave me great pain,' she had written when she thought he was still alive. But he had died of AIDS, in Melbourne, Australia, aged 33, and John Foster had buried him in Kew Cemetery. 'Sacred to the memory of Juan Gualberto Céspedes' were the improbable words inscribed on Gosford sandstone, in that countrified suburban place of the dead.

But it is not by any means a funereal account of a life

that Foster unfolds, even though the story of Juan's last days is very affecting. Juan was a sickly child, scarcely at home in Castro's Cuba, a blithe and lyrical dancer who left the National Ballet School there under some sort of cloud. 'Johnny,' he would say to Foster in Manhattan, 'I didn't do *nothing*!'

He seems to have been a creature of grace, child-like but full of attitude, leaving a deep impression on those he touched, however lightly. Shakespeare says somewhere that he's a fool who trusts in a boy's love and the Juan who rises from Foster's pages as a great tragicomic figure was always a boy it seems, though the book Foster has written is a book of wisdom that does its subject proud. After his death one of his old boyfriends wrote to Foster from New York, 'I sense from your account … that many people are increased in their humanity because of Juan's presence among them.'

The logic of this wholly unsentimental book is to persuade us how this might have been so. It works because Foster has effected an extraordinary imaginative glow which somehow bathes the figure of Juan; for all his petulance and extravagance he is treated with a subtlety and richness, a play of light and dark, normally reserved for characters in the upper levels of fiction.

We follow Juan through a summary of the rattiness of his New York existence (tawdry and magnificent, by turns) among the spirited queens striving to get by. Foster negotiates this life of Juan before the life he shared with him with sure-footedness and narrative grace, exhibiting a writerly assurance few novelists can match.

If someone else, some stranger, were telling Juan's story, I expect their chapter might finish here, at the very nadir of his fortunes. That would accord with Juan's own sense of things, and give due weight to the crucial event. And it would restore a fairer balance, some better proportion to the recollections of his life; because already it was more than two-thirds spent.

But this story is also my story, and has my memory's shape. And so it continues, relating all those things that happened in New York before we met. Before we began to join our lives.

This looks like the technique of fiction, this cadenced prose with its air of impending fatality, but its predetermined effects are not only the facts of Foster's life, they are also something he never presumes on (or fails to recreate), such is the artistry of his narrative. Passages like this sound reminiscent of the David Malouf of *Johnno*, which some of us think is his best book, but Foster has a story which is not only true but which is erotically unashamed and indisputably calamitous. It would be ridiculous to style this as an advantage but his book will certainly bear comparison with Malouf's. Indeed in its sustained elegance, its relative freedom of form and its easy command of dialogue and anecdote as well as in its absolute credibility, it can sometimes seem superior.

The coming together of the two men is done sparely and without excessive emphasis and there is no mawkishness through the stages of emotional delineation. They determine to go back to Australia together, though the narrative manages to sustain its electricity through Juan's various, more or less drama queen-like reactions, to the difficulties and humiliations that befall him as he follows Foster around Britain and Europe. Throughout the depiction of all this Foster shows remarkable command of tempo and an effortless ability to keep his characterisations vivid. This descriptive prose gleans with the skills of a natural scene-painter, a born travel writer with a potentially virtuoso technique in the manner of Patrick Leigh Fermor who nevertheless has the very un-Australian virtue of restraint, a man who is content to show what language can do rather than what can be done with language.

> I flew into New York with the snow. Five years earlier, on my first visit, I had detested the worn-out February snow, packed hard and piss-stained where a thousand dogs had walked their owners on the streets. It had seemed like a two-toned city, yellow and grey like the ribbons that had still been fastened to the street trees to celebrate the release of the Middle East hostages and the end of the '444 days of degradation'.

Foster is a sharp-witted stylist, sparing of his own and anyone else's linguistic jewels. The last movement of the book, from the moment when Juan is diagnosed as HIV-positive until his death, has enormous concentration and dramatic punch, though it is everywhere enlivened by perceptions which are on the verge of being tart. An officious doctor forces the homosexual couple to think of last things when she says, 'I want to talk to you about AIDS … It will help you to plan your lives,' and Foster reflects, 'Was she pronouncing a sentence of death already?' and later, when the end is near, he thinks with something close to hatred of Juan having to confront the TV image of the Grim Reaper ('this fantastic cowled creature, socket-eyed and scythe-swinging') as he lies on his actual deathbed.

Throughout the never simply sombre description of these last days, poignant with Juan's reiterated fear of dying, there are vivid snatches that dramatise the situation, visually and complexly, within a social field – as when he appears at a dance in his old New York fur coat or when he hears himself named among the sick for whom prayers are offered on Palm Sunday – which he insists on attending in the Anglican church they both frequent – and says hearing his name, quite audibly, 'Take away this pain.'

There are moments of comedy in the midst of blackness and moments of black comedy. And indeed, much of what makes this book such a magnificent piece of writing is its refusal to gainsay the terrible quality of what happened. 'And then, most cruelly, in a way that I found unbearable he was assaulted, battered with the idea of death.' That's Foster's description of the Grim Reaper on TV. Juan tells him not to turn it off. It won't last long, he says.

The deathbed scenes are remarkable, not least for the depiction of this dying bird of paradise achieving patience in the midst of it all – it being fear of death and of futility. 'Out of that patience', Foster writes, 'came the greatest sadness, a sadness that lodged in me it seems for ever …'

And then at last, more than a year later, there is the journeying to Cuba, to the mother who had said, 'I hardly remember your face but I hope to embrace you before I die.'

It should be clear that I have a high opinion of *Take Me to Paris, Johnny*. It is a memoir which yields nothing to fiction in the imagination it displays and in the power and sweep of the emotions it depicts and conveys. Indeed it makes most fiction, here or elsewhere, look paltry by comparison. This is a book full of the accents of comedy which is nevertheless as tragic as an intimate account of everyday life can be. It is a book full of intelligence and laughter which is also deeply – never depressingly – sad. It's difficult to imagine a reader who will not feel in John Foster's debt.

Peter Craven

CHAPTER ONE

Nobody knew what the crime was but it seemed at the time
that it was something inherent, like being a Jew in Germany
around 1936. The country, it is true, was poor in Jews but rich
in *maricones, patos, pájaros, cundangos, locas,* and *pederastas*: the
nomenclator's paradise.

—G. Cabrera Infante, *View of Dawn in the Tropics*

From Santiago de Cuba the road ran east through the
central valley of the province. The country was exactly as I
wanted it to be—red earth, banana plantations and hills that
were crowned with a darker canopy of royal palms. Across
the rising terrain to the north lay the Sierra del Cristal
where Fidel Castro's brother had opened up the second
front of the Revolution. Ahead, beyond the hills, were the
Atlantic beaches of Baracoa where Columbus once claimed
the island for the Spanish Crown. In the cathedral of that
town—so they say—is preserved the cross that he planted in
the sand. Later, when it was encased in precious metals and
exposed to the veneration of the faithful, it brought them
good fortune. Or, to put the matter more circumspectly, it
rendered their fortunes less evil than they might otherwise

have been. This was no mean blessing, for it is difficult to conceive how they could have borne more suffering than they did endure: slavery, revolt and civil war. Since the triumph of the Revolution, according to my driver, the efficacy of the cross had declined. By what measure this diminished power was established he did not say, and I reflected privately that in matters of unbelief a certain scepticism was required.

I never reached the legendary regions of the mountains and the sea. My destination was the city of Guantánamo. It was also afflicted with fame, more recently acquired, and acknowledged by Fidel when he bestowed on it the honorific title 'First Trench of the Revolution'. Foremost among the cities of Cuba, it held the front line against imperialism, which maintained a toehold here in the form of the American naval base.

I hope the Guantanamerans were grateful for this sign of recognition. Their town had few other claims to distinction. As we approached the outskirts the landscape took on a desolate air; it was brown, scarred and smudged with a confusion of railway marshalling yards, the end of the line. Even my guidebook (which was written with the assistance of the National Tourism Institute and could not be accused of false objectivity) conceded that Guantánamo remained extremely underdeveloped and that its improvement would require many years of concentrated revolutionary effort.

During the bourgeois era things had been different, though not necessarily better. Then everything had revolved around the naval base which the Americans had established in 1902 to guarantee Cuba's hard-won independence from Spain. A city built on slavery adjusted easily to the requirements and opportunities of the new order; the buying and selling of human flesh continued, except that now it was paid for by American servicemen. Compared with the wild oscillations of the international sugar market to which the fortunes of the town had always been tied, the American trade was laudably regular and dependable. And so a flourishing prostitution business arose and was passed down from one generation to another like titles to land.

The base created other jobs which, though less lucrative, were less offensive to the honour of the nation. One of these was held, when the border was still open in the days of the dictator Batista, by the baker Céspedes. He was, as far as I know, an estimable and patriotic man who drank no more than his share of beer and rum. He baked the Americans' bread without reproach and then, with equal skill, he baked the bread for the Revolution. 'Freedom with bread; bread without terror!' Fidel had proclaimed, and when the slogan went up on hoardings all over the country, it must have been good for the baker's business. He had no complaints about the Revolution.

It was the baker Céspedes, or more precisely his wife, whom I had come to see. I located the address on the Calle Pinto in a long, low row of houses between San Lino and Santa Rita. All along the whitewashed terrace windows were shuttered against the sun; behind them, and from the half-open doorways, watched a hundred pairs of eyes, grateful for any diversion from the boredom of the afternoon. Children playing in the road stopped their game and stared. A gang of youths, too cool to betray their curiosity openly, continued to fan their bellies with the bottom of their T-shirts and observed me with sidelong glances. In New York my expatriate friends had told me that I should not come. Fidel, they said, had more eyes than a peacock's tail.

The whole town would know I was there, and no good could come of it for the family. Be content with your memories, they said.

But still I had to come, driven to seek out this poor house, poorer than I had ever imagined. The sight of it confused me, and yet it was strangely exhilarating to be walking on this street, about to knock on this door. It was too late to turn back now.

A woman appeared on the doorstep: mid-fifties, greying hair, wearing a red cotton print dress. If she was the person in the snapshot, she had put on weight. I was unsure.

'Señora Gomez?'

'Si.'

'La madre de Juan?'

I had imagined this meeting many times, prepared my script, rehearsed the Spanish phrases. But the mention of his name and the sight of my foreign face told her all she needed to know. She paused, and then she was on the pavement, hugging me, her face buried on my shoulder, her horn-rimmed spectacles pressing into my collar-bone. She was crying.

She had known about Juan's illness. In his letters he had told her, as he told anyone who bothered to enquire about the state of his health, that he had an ulcer. Early in 1986, in the absence of a definite medical diagnosis, that had seemed a reasonable explanation of his persistent stomach pains, and there had been no point in canvassing any more sinister alternative.

She had replied promptly to the first intimation of this news. 'Son, I tell you that I very much regret you have a stomach ulcer but I advise you to look after yourself and don't do stupid things like eating spicy food since this is

4

very dangerous. Carry out the treatment as the doctor has told you.'

In a subsequent letter he must have tried to allay her concern. There was, after all, no ulcer. Nevertheless, she continued to fret maternally. In December she had urged him to find a tablet or a medicine so this would not happen again. In the name of God and of all the saints and of St Barbara she hoped that he would be well. 'The only desire in my life', she had written, 'is to be able to see you one day with all my soul because you were my son. I hardly remember your face, but I hope to embrace you and kiss you one day before I die.'

After this there had been silence from Cuba, most likely because she was waiting for a reply that never came. Finally, nearly six months later she had written again:

17 June
Year 29 of the Revolution

My dear son,

Before anything else a strong embrace and a big kiss that will touch the heart of us both.

I have an immense desire to see you but it appears that destiny does not want it that way. I carry you in my heart and bless you every day so that things will work out as you want.

I must tell you that on Mothers' Day I received no word from you which gave me great pain.

It was not her son who opened that letter, not the son whose face she scarcely remembered, whom destiny had removed from her embrace. It was I who opened the letter, which made it clear that she had not received the news that I had sent in April. Why not? The mail to Cuba was slow, but it could hardly take eight weeks. Had some sharp-eyed postal clerk spotted the letter and steamed off the exotic stamps? Or had the censor intervened?

'Did you never receive my letter?' I asked, when we were sitting in the living-room of the low white house. 'It was a long letter, several pages, in good Spanish that my neighbour from Peru translated for me.'

'No,' she said. 'From Australia I heard nothing. I heard only from Germany.'

After her Mothers' Day letter I had decided to write to Juan's younger brother Rafi in East Germany so that he could relay the message from there. With such delicacy as I could command, I had sent him the news that his brother was dead. He had died of AIDS, but since I did not know (though I could well imagine) how that sickness might be regarded in Cuba, I had not included this detail in my letter to his mother which, in any case, it seemed that she had not received. And so it was from Weimar that the news finally reached the house on the Calle Pinto.

Now, after the passage of a year, I unpacked the few mementos I had brought with me: a pair of ballet shoes that had been tucked together at the bottom of a suitcase, a handful of photos, and a picture of the grave. For the tombstone the mason had suggested a black marble that could be polished to a mirror finish. 'It lasts forever,' he had said; 'Specially imported. From South Africa.' That meant that it was out of the question. Instead, I had sent to Sydney for a supply of Gosford sandstone, and on that more friendly surface were engraved the words:

✠

Sacred to the Memory

of

JUAN GUALBERTO CÉSPEDES

BORN 12 JULY 1953

IN CUBA

DIED 17 APRIL 1987

Sitting in her wicker chair, his mother gazed at the photo and said nothing. Her face was closed. Was she trying to decipher the Gothic lettering of the first line? The mason thought this flourish gave the inscription a touch of class, but it seemed to me merely sentimental, and I regretted not having instructed him more carefully. Unnerved by so much concentrated silence, or simply distracted by this curious intervention in the routine of his retirement, the baker Céspedes—who was also present—opened the bottle of rum I had brought from the dollar shop in Santiago. He was hunting for a glass when she said, without looking up, 'But of *what* did he die?'

In this gravestone she was confronted again with the evasiveness in which Juan had shrouded his life and which she had tried so often, and so unsuccessfully, to penetrate in her letters. 'Write to me telling me how you are, but do not send me a letter telling me lies, because I want to know the truth of your life.' From her restricted perspective nothing in his life had seemed fixed. 'Do you live in America or Australia?' she had asked in genuine bewilderment. But if Juan had not told her, and Rafi would not, neither was it for me to tell her the truth of his death. It was enough to say that he had died of a virus for which they could find no remedy.

There was one last memento: a copy of John Rickard's book *Australia: A Cultural History*, which had been launched just before I left for Cuba. It was written with a foreign readership in mind, though hardly so foreign, I imagine, as the audience it found here in Guantánamo. What would a Cuban reader make of Dame Edna Everage, portrayed here kicking up her outsize feet on the desk of the editor of *Quadrant*? It didn't matter. In this shuttered room on the Calle Pinto the pictures of Mr Chifley gazing into the prototypical jaws of a Holden sedan, of Bondi beach boys indulging themselves, of Billy Graham crusading for Christ in heathen Sydney—all these were no more than footnotes to the clean white page of the dedication. It was for Juan and me. This was the only public place in which our names appeared together, the next best thing to a marriage notice, I thought, as though there were no grave that intervened. And in this dedication, I persuaded myself, she might see more clearly what before she could only have surmised.

For a moment she disappeared into the other room, and came back with a children's picture book that had been recycled as a photo album. This, it transpired, contained the meagre record of Juan's life: three childhood portraits, all slightly defiant—prettily, sourly, doggedly—as though he were determined to reject the blame that had vaguely attached to him since his difficult birth.

He was born in July 1953, at the beginning of Carnival. Two weeks after he had made his troublesome entry into the world, there was another sign that this was an inauspicious month for new beginnings. Only a few miles away to the west, while the country partied and drank itself to a standstill, Fidel Castro and his band of guerrillas launched their famous attack on the Moncada barracks. It was to have been the signal for revolt, a call to the nation to enlist against the dictatorship under the banner of liberty. It failed, and the rebels were hunted down like dogs. When one of their number refused to divulge the secrets of the group, she was presented with the gouged-out eyes of her brother. When she refused again, she was offered the testicles of her lover. That was in July 1953, at the end of Carnival, in the month that Juan was born.

Fidel was captured and arraigned before the judge. He rejected any guilt: 'History will absolve me,' he told the judge. But history, to which Fidel appealed with the confidence of one who intended to make it, absolves (or condemns) only those who cut a figure in the world. Mostly it neither absolves nor condemns; it simply forgets.

Without a special claim on history, Juan would have to depend for absolution on the more conventional rites and capacious memory of the church. His grandmother saw to that. She presented him for baptism at the parish church of Santa Catarina de Ricci who, appropriately for a town with such inadequate sanitation, specialised in the cure of stomach complaints. The mystical washing away of his sin, one may reasonably assume, was satisfactorily accomplished. The expiation of his guilt was not. For it arose, after all, not so much from his fault as from the fault that was imputed to him.

The fault grew. He became that most provoking phenomenon, a delicate child whose condition neither worsened nor improved, who neither flourished nor sickened. He required and received from his grandmother special attention, and they entered accordingly into a conspiracy of affection. When his stomach revolted against cow's milk, or powdered milk, or tins of American milk, Clara de la Rosa pressed him fresh guava juice. When he would not eat for fear of his bowels running, she fried him sweet white fish for breakfast. When there was rice, his must come from the bottom of the pan where it was allowed to catch on the fire and crisp in just the right degree.

And then, five years and five months after her first difficult birth, when the doctor had told her she might never have another child, Juan's mother was delivered of a second son. Uncomplicated, healthy Rafi bounced into the world under the star of the Revolution, in the very month of the Triumph. His arrival compounded Juan's guilt. He would always be measured against his younger brother and often be found wanting. Neither flight nor the passage of years would release him from the expectations that pressed on him as the older son. Even twenty-five years later his mother would write:

> Do you still love me now that Rafael is big? This is to tell you that I need you, if you can, to help me. I have been making a house for more than five years and I cannot finish it because of the economic situation. I need you to send me some money, and I ask you this as your mother because I truly need it. Reply urgently so that I know whether I can count on you, or whether your brother will have to start work and leave his studies.

In the matter of the house, which involved the construction of a third room, Juan did what little he could. With the punitive exchange rate and the government levy the dollars he sent were reduced to a pitifully small number of pesos. But the arrival even of a small amount of money in

10

Guantánamo made news. In other, paler parts of the country, from which the white middle classes had fled the Revolution in their hundreds of thousands, parcels and remittances from Miami and New Jersey were commonplace. From black Guantánamo, though, there had been few refugees. This town had been solid for Fidel from the beginning. '*Patria o muerte!*' they had cried, an admirable sentiment so long as it was not put to the test. And besides, what attraction could there be for them in the United States where black people, as they had heard, were lynched? But patriotism and pride had an unanticipated disadvantage, and the consequence was that in this part of the country there were few remittances from abroad.

It is understandable, therefore, that when work began on the third room of the Céspedes house, it excited comment. Especially it stirred deep memories in a younger neighbour, one Tania, who determined to apply to Juan's mother for his address. How sweetly she must have talked, how nostalgically she yearned to renew an old friendship! And how pleased she was to receive his address!

'I'm earning 110 pesos to maintain three boys and I cannot lift my head,' she wrote to her *querido y estimado amigo Juan*.

He who has nothing is looked down upon. I know that—you for me and I for you—we are like brothers since our childhood. If I have not written to you earlier, don't call me false. Juan Gualberto, I know it is within your reach because some friends of mine have been sent to. I do not need anything else; only a cheque for 500 dollars to buy clothes for these boys. Do not send goods because I cannot redeem the parcel from the post office.

11

A letter from Cuba always meant drama. There would sometimes be tears, sometimes a morose, impenetrable silence as he worked his way again through layers of regret and loneliness. This, though, produced a flash of fury that settled into brooding anger. The temerity of the woman outraged him. How could he ever forget the way she had made his teenage years a misery? She had hounded him, tormented him, branded him as a faggot. And now, incredibly, she came begging for five hundred dollars.

She had called him a faggot, a *loca*, a queen, a crazy one—not once, I suspect, but repeatedly, with that particular venom that teenage girls can so devastatingly deploy. Each time she taunted him she pronounced a sentence of excommunication, as surely as if she had been the Bishop of Havana himself. Or you might say she spoke with the power of those triumphant guerrillas with their adorable revolutionary beards who set before the country new and higher standards of *machismo*. Or perhaps she spoke only for her disappointed adolescent self. Whatever the case, the result was the same. A *loca* was ridiculous, no more than a village idiot in drag.

And, of course, it was true. Why else, all those years ago, had her dear and esteemed Juan Gualberto sauntered off in the evenings to join the little gaggle of youths who assembled in *el Parque 24*, or on the square in front of the cemetery on the edge of town, or in the bushes that grew along the Guantánamo River? In these out-of-the-way places he had discovered a circle of friends, an amusing and special society where the queenly figure of La Negra held court. She was a handsome youth, slim and spectacularly black, and she knew how to enhance the impact she made. She could flutter her made-up eyelashes with fatal charm; she could toss her straightened black hair with Hollywood panache. By comparison, her companions were rather less chic. There was Tomasa Corduroy, whom the Revolution had unfairly restricted to the one pair of trousers from which she derived her name. And La Bizca, in whom one eye crossed the other when she was angry or excited, a decided misfortune, though to a connoisseur it might have an unpredictable attraction.

In this company Juan Gualberto was also transformed. 'Such a noisy boy,' La Negra recalled. 'So loud.' But he had pretensions to elegance. Within this charming circle he took on the neatly androgynous name of Michel(le), to which, with impressive *hauteur*, he attached the surname D'Ambreville. They were names from his grandmother's family, bestowed originally by a French plantation owner on the Haitian slave from whom Clara de la Rosa was descended. Those were the names he chose, assuming at once the identity of a slave and an aristocrat. He might be a faggot, but he would not be common.

Nevertheless, he was a scandal. The fault in him was visible. At home he could still rely on his grandmother for moral support, though when he danced about or acted queenishly, even she would join in poking fun at him: '*La puta in acción!*' For the baker Céspedes it was past a joke. With commendable fatherly concern he began to enquire whether there was not a chance of placing such a talented boy as his in a scholarship programme in Havana. It happened that there was. No doubt the baker agreed that one could not be too particular in choosing a career; one had to consider the needs of the Revolution as well as the opportunities it presented. In this way Juan found himself enrolled in the Veterinary Institute Juan P. Carbo Servia. And in a time-honoured way a small-town family relieved itself of an unmerited embarrassment.

It may be that I have done the baker an injustice. About these events Juan was singularly silent. But it is true to say that the veterinary career on which he so surprisingly embarked never fired his imagination.

Nor, it seems, did Havana itself. Why, I wondered, when I came to wander through the streets of the old city and along the great sea wall, did he never hint at the fabulous faded beauty of this city? A thirteen-year-old scholarship student cannot be expected to enthuse about the glories of colonial architecture or the patterning of glass in the fanlights of a palace courtyard. But did he not recall the dappled shade of the Prado where the wives of Spanish merchants, and then the high-class prostitutes, had once paraded in the evening breeze? Or the banks of gardenias around the white marble fountain in the *Parque Central*? He never referred to these things; and if I mention them now, it is because I like to invest his memory with their fragrances.

Juan's Havana was crystallised, set and polished in one recurring image. In Guantánamo he had taken dancing lessons, and his aptitude was such that when he arrived in Havana to study goats and cows he was also admitted to classes with the school of the National Ballet. The revolutionary credentials of this institution were impeccable. Alicia Alonso had founded it in 1948. She had gone into exile under the dictatorship, and she returned after the Triumph to establish an art not of kings and of rulers but rather an art of the people. And was not the scholarship boy from Guantánamo of the people? Even if, as he noticed, the people at the ballet were almost entirely white? So why did they come to him—sometime in 1968—with the objection that though he danced like an angel and had great talent, he was not quite suitable for the school? His conduct, they managed to imply, was not quite proper. He would have to leave. The injustice of it stunned him. In the fog of words he heard again the taunting voice of Tania. His protests went unheard. 'Johnny,' he told me a dozen times, 'I didn't do *nothing!*'

That was precisely the point. It was puzzling only if you assumed, as he most certainly had, that they judged you on the basis of your actions. What he had not yet learned was that the Revolution took a broader view of a man. Of course it was interested in what you did, and the Committees for its Defence kept a careful watch on that. (Is this what the poet meant by 'loving the Revolution's impact on the eyes'?) But it was also curious to know what you *were*, so that it might more efficiently determine what you would become.

This was no ordinary revolution. It aimed at nothing less than the reformation of the human race. Society, said El Che, must be converted into a gigantic school, a vast reformatory. The Maximum Leader agreed. And so the great experiment began, to the plaudits of French philosophers, American radicals and liberal churchmen who flocked to the island paradise to witness the realisation of a dream, and to savour the paradox that was Cuba: so slow to abolish slavery, so late to overthrow the Spanish yoke, yet now the cradle of the future, the birthplace of the New Man.

The shortcomings of the old model were evident enough. Fidel recited them with ready facility, which was a tribute to his orderly Jesuit education: egoism, greed, sensuality, sloth, prostitution of all sorts, usury. These, according to El Che, were the ways of wolves. The New Man, stripped of petit-bourgeois morality and ideology, would govern his conduct by 'the most noble principles of collectivism, self-sacrifice, love of work, hatred of exploitation and parasitism, and a fraternal spirit of co-operation and solidarity'.

Inspired by this splendid vision, the Revolution went to work with a will. At first the Chief of Public Order made the battle against petit-bourgeois decadence his personal responsibility. With his men he would surround the *posadas* of Havana with lights and loud-hailers and announce: 'You have five minutes from now to abandon your vicious antics!' Such were the demands of this crusade that the Chief himself became exhausted and retired to a less strenuous existence in the United States. The campaign, however, went on. The stream of sexual tourists dried up. Parasitism declined. The gay bars of Havana—the San Michel, the Dirty Dick and sundry other stains on the national honour—were swept away. And yet tell-tale signs of the old order persisted. In particular, it appeared that sterner measures were needed to eliminate the sickness, *la enfermedad*, of unnatural desire. This infirmity was discovered in the most exalted places: in the ministries of state, in the University, in the Union of Artists and Writers. Detected cases were systematically removed, and a watchful eye was kept on the dangerous professions that were so unaccountably prone to infection. In due course the watchful eye extended its gaze to the school of the National Ballet, and there it lighted on the suspect figure of the dancing Juan.

The most noble principle of collectivism dictated that he should be removed, and the health of the Ballet was thus protected. But as he was only fourteen, his own cure was deferred until the malady had fully ripened. The Revolution could be patient, and so he had time to contemplate his future treatment. What form it might take he learned

16

from La Negra, who had been an early beneficiary of the programme.

Her treatment had begun quite unexpectedly, at the time of the annual military call-up. On the appointed day she had reported, as required, in the town square, along with the other conscripts of her year. A sergeant sorted them according to their various intended destinations. La Negra had indicated to the authorities a preference for the airforce, which seemed more stylish than the army. But strangely, she found herself allotted to a company of curiously unmilitary types: sons of the swinish rich, a priest, a pimp and a poofter. Soldiers with bayonets prodded them into the back of a truck. 'Hardly the way to treat your new recruits,' she thought. And then, as they left the city and rolled north across the country to the province of Camaguey, the treatment began.

When they arrived at their camp, the staff assembled to greet them. They were ordered to undress. They were issued with grey shirts, green fatigues and working boots—'the lowest class in the lowest echelon of shoes'. They were taken to a football field, given a total haircut and set to work cutting cane. They had been recruited, they now realised, to a Military Unit to Aid Production. In other countries and at other times the UMAPs, as they were called, were more simply known as concentration camps. And so it was appropriate that there was a large sign above the entrance gate which said: WORK WILL MAKE A MAN OF YOU!

Of course, a man is not made by work alone. For that, education is also necessary, which is why the camp provided classes for instruction in the principles of the Revolution. At first these classes were co-educational, so to speak, but then it appeared that the *locas* had a curious knack of subverting

17

the learning process, so they were given separate attention and helped to learn with beatings. A couple went crazy; a couple killed themselves; a few escaped.

La Negra's treatment lasted for two years until one day, when she could no longer stand on her swollen feet, and with infected lungs, unexpectedly they sent her home. The treatment had failed, but at least it had confirmed the initial diagnosis. She was indeed an invalid.

By the time La Negra returned to Guantánamo, the Revolution was nearly ten years old. The Year of the Heroic Guerrilla had drawn to a close and the Year of the Decisive Effort had dawned. Fidel was rallying the nation again, this time in aid of the sadly underdeveloped economy. The Revolution needed cash, and to secure it, the energy of the whole people must be harnessed to achieve a sugar harvest of unprecedented magnitude: ten million tons! They should work, urged Fidel (who was growing increasingly fond of military metaphors) like soldiers in the face of an enemy attack. Nothing should interfere with their will to battle. Even Christmas, and the Feast of the Three Kings, was postponed for six months until the harvest could be safely gathered in.

The scholarship students, too, were required to participate in the intended triumph of the record harvest. One of them, a girl from Guantánamo, was interviewed by a team of American anthropologists who happened to be in Cuba at the time.

> Of course [she told them] things are going to be just a little bit scarcer now, because all the workers are spending so much time in the sugar cane harvest so we can finally stop being an underdeveloped country and

18

strike yet another blow against imperialism. We're determined that Cuba shall remain sovereign and free, that never again shall a traitor trample it underfoot. My fatherland comes first with me. I'd rather die than see it under the imperialist yoke.

Fatherland or death! *Patria o muerte!* How correct she was, this girl. She thought a lot about the future. 'Nothing is impossible now,' she told the anthropologists. 'Whatever I propose to do, I can.' Writing was her vocation: 'writing perhaps about the Revolution, so that future generations will know how we lived. That's my dream and I know that some day I'll wake up and find it come true.'

When Juan Gualberto contemplated his future in that decisive year, it must have appeared less enticing: ten million tons of sugar; and then back to the dreary routine of the Veterinary Institute of Havana where they were making him learn Russian. After that, when he would finally come of military age, a concentration camp.

In making this sombre assessment of his prospects, his view was undoubtedly coloured by that bourgeois individualism that the Party so strongly deplored. As the watchful eye at the Ballet School had foreseen, the fault in him that had first shown up as a mere lack of manliness was beginning to bear its ideological fruit. He was developing counter-revolutionary tendencies. He murmured against the sacrificial shortages, against the monotonous ration of rice soup and the nauseous macaroni. He hated his one pair of white cotton trousers which, at the end of a day in the harvest, were stiff as a board from the dried juice of the sugar cane. He despised the red-faced Russians he had observed in the streets of Havana and hated their grating language.

No wonder, then, that back home for the Year of Decisive Effort, he was more charmed than ever by the forbidden music from the radio station at the navy base. No wonder that he idolised the Supremes, that he memorised the lyrics of Dionne Warwick; that he dreamed, still, of dancing; that he was excited by the talk he heard in the little queenly circle that met, though now more furtively, at the edge of the cemetery.

As the very correct girl had told the anthropologists, nothing is impossible. If the Revolution would not accommodate your dreams, so much the worse for the Revolution. Cuba might be a prison, but it was not escape-proof. Everybody knew that. There had been many fugitives, and many deaths as the refugees launched themselves in leaking boats and rafts on the current that would float them, they prayed, to Florida. But in Guantánamo there was a more tempting possibility—the short but hazardous route across the border to the US naval base.

When she had recovered sufficiently from her treatment, La Negra was among the first to take this route; and when it was clear that she had made good her escape, others prepared to follow. Then it was time for Juan.

Did he leave defiantly? With mock bravado? Or sick with fear, not least the fear of losing face if he pulled back at the last moment? I know only that he left silently, without farewells, in the company of an older friend called Alex.

At night they made their way to the coast near the border, slipping past the watchtower when the guards changed duty. By day they hid in a mangrove swamp. Then in the darkness of the second night they made their way through the salt flats that stretched into the sea and struck out, half stumbling and half swimming, across the water to the base. A boat picked them up in its searchlight. There was shouting, but in the humid June night the voices did not carry. They could see no insignia. The boat drew alongside and fished them out of the sea. And thank God, said Juan when he recited this story as a party trick, it was the Americans!

At the naval base they were accorded the status of political refugees and then despatched to Miami to join a bunch of other escapees in the care of a Catholic refugee agency. When they had been properly processed, they were asked about their intended destination. Some chose to stay in Florida, others nominated Los Angeles or Chicago. Then they came to Juan. 'Take me to Paris!' he said. They did the best they could, and put him on the train to New York City.

He was free, and fifteen, and he had stored up for himself an agony of future remorse. How could he have known, as he travelled north, that he had broken the heart of Clara de la Rosa? Or that his mother would give birth ten months later to a second brother whom he would never see.

CHAPTER TWO

Life is no dream! Beware and beware and beware!
We tumble downstairs to eat the damp of the earth
Or we climb to the snowy divide with the choir
of dead dahlias,
But neither dream nor forgetfulness is:
Brute flesh is.

—Garcia Lorca, 'Sleepless City'

Many years later Juan Gualberto composed a fragment of autobiography. Strictly speaking, it was a *curriculum vitae*, and as it was intended for the eyes of a government minister, it was necessarily economical with facts.

'When I arrived in New York,' it began. He didn't say, and the minister hardly needed to know, that when he arrived in New York the city was grotesquely unlike anything he had anticipated. Wall-to-wall hippies, he remembered, when he cast his mind back to the summer of 1969. Vietnam vets returning; and drugs, so many drugs that these Americans seemed to be brain-damaged, drugged to their ears, tripping, crashing and over-dosing. This at least was how it looked from Hell's Kitchen, where the Catholic agency had installed its Cuban refugees in a cheap apartment house. The other residents, according to Juan's calculation, consisted of 25 per cent ex-cons, 25 per cent drag queens and 50 per cent addicts.

Outside this depressing neighbourhood, on 42nd Street, he liked the lights and the crowds. And over on Times Square, where the grid of streets tied itself into a concentrated knot of energy, he was awed by the sheer profusion of the scene. You could go bowling here, and roll rubber balls into slots in a pokerina parlour, and watch flapjacks being flipped on a window grill. There was a shop where you could buy a Swiss hat with your name stitched in it, and another where they analysed you by computer. Best of all you could watch the ebb and flow of the crowds, day and night, eating, spending, touring, cruising and loving the mass spectacle of their massed selves.

Had he ventured further afield on those first two nights in Manhattan, he might have seen a still more memorable spectacle. There were riots on those nights in a Greenwich Village pub. The Stonewall Inn was frequented by homosexuals, and was periodically raided by the police. But on this occasion the homosexuals decided that they had had enough of this kind of treatment. So Juan could have said, 'I came in'—that was the phrase he always used to describe his arrival in New York—'I came in with Gay Liberation.'

He didn't say that; but what he did say was equally arresting. He came in with the man on the moon. It was an awesome climax, that moon landing, to a fabulous summer: Woodstock, Stonewall, and then the moon. All over the country people were glued to their TV screens. It was a triumph of the human spirit, a feat of American technology, and much else besides, though there were some, according to a survey conducted by the *Times*, who couldn't have cared less. But Juan cared, passionately. He watched it all on an open-air screen in Times Square.

'Do you remember', I once asked him, 'what you thought when you watched the landing?'

'Yes,' he smiled back, 'how Fidel must be biting his tail!'

How would he find his way, who could he be in this place that dizzied him with such conflicting impressions: fear, contempt, exhilaration and a strong dose of self-vindicating *Schadenfreude*? He needed a guide, an interpreter. And so it was of more than casual significance that his account to the Minister began with an encounter.

> When I arrived in New York [he wrote], I met Father E.B. He found me a school to learn English. I also began to take private dance lessons. In the summer of 1970 I auditioned for the Harkness Ballet and was accepted; and in September of the same year I was accepted as well with the Joffrey Ballet. From then on my goal in life was to be a dancer and I gave it my complete attention.

How did he meet this exemplary priest? Juan, I suspect, would have found the question of no interest. In New York City, as he described it, you simply bumped into people; they careered towards you out of the crowd with an air of fatality in a way that could neither be foreseen nor deflected. So the priest, when he appeared, required no explanation, although in retrospect one might see in him the first instalment of Juan's own particular method of managing the American dream.

In short, he had found a patron. The affection and

guidance that the priest provided were not entirely disinterested, but it would be churlish to esteem him less highly on this account. He was generous; with his time, his money, his house, his table and his bed. And if Juan had any cause for complaint, it was at first nothing more serious than the under-developed culinary imagination of his benefactor. A Cuban, he thought, should not be required to exist on a perpetual diet of steak and salad. After two or three days with the priest at his rectory in Greenwich Village, he was always glad to return to the apartment he shared with Alex on 103rd Street, where there would be a proper meal of rice and chicken and beans.

For two years, or possibly three, this agreeable arrangement persisted until, in ways so vague, so undefinable that Juan was never able to recall with any clarity, the relationship began to sour. Perhaps the priest was tiring of his young protégé, finding his charms too easy, his tastes too expensive or his occasional tantrums too exhausting. Or it may be that he was piqued by the attention that his boy was able to attract, and respond to, in the gay clubs that he was beginning to frequent. Whatever the reason, there came a parting of the ways: angry, ugly, and construed by Juan as betrayal.

He condensed the tawdry details into the memory of two incidents. The first happened one night when he went out with the priest to a restaurant in the Village. It was an event so commonplace, so trivial, that it is surprising to reflect that the ripples of it touched my own life more than a decade later, and extended even to the desk of the Minister for Immigration in Canberra. In the restaurant a waiter brought them a basket of bread, and the bread, when they opened it, was host to a nest of cockroaches. You did not have to be a Manhattan sophisticate to resent being served a tribe of insects for your dinner. Yet in the opinion of the restaurateur that was no justification for the violent row that ensued, for the escalating frenzy of insults and the wild overturning of the table. The police, when they came, agreed with the restaurateur, and the priest, in his embarrassment, agreed with the police, so that Juan was charged with disorderly conduct. It was, of course, unfair, which the court recognised when it heard the charge, but the magistrate gave him a lecture anyhow on the need to control his Latin temper.

About the betrayal of the priest they said nothing. Yet this was what burnt itself in Juan's memory, and he remembered it because, in those days between the cockroaches and the court, he lived in terror, in gut-wrenching fear that they would deport him, return him to the mercies of the Revolution that he had deserted. Surely that could not have been what the priest intended?

Soon after the episode with the cockroaches he finally parted company with his patron. The occasion he once again remembered in the context of a meal. Although it was of no moment to Juan, who adopted a thoroughly ecumenical spirit in his relationships, it happened that the priest was of the Episcopalian persuasion. This meant not only that he could marry but, in the opinion of a New England aunt who appears to have borne some family responsibility for her clerical nephew, that he should. Had she heard that his ministry in the Village was giving rise to scandal? Whatever her motives may have been, she arranged a luncheon at which Juan also contrived to be present, and there she pressed the claims of marriage on her nephew. Certainly, she considered, even in the absence of a suitable girl, the 'Cuban boy' would have to go, and a savage, speechless, retaliatory

Cuban kick on the shins (which he always remembered with grim satisfaction) did nothing to alter her absolute resolve.

An aunt like this will have her way. And it may indeed have been a way that the priest himself desired, lured to the prospect of marriage by the siren manipulation of his therapist who, I imagine, promised him an integrated personality if he would only direct his energies to a real woman. In any event the boy was dismissed, and in due course the priest entered on a more conventional exercise of his sacred vocation, supported by the comfort of a wife in a Connecticut rectory.

Although in the end Juan fought with the priest like a wild cat, there had been a time, at least for a while, when the priest had believed in him, in his talent and in his future. He had paid the fees for the private dancing lessons that opened the way to the Joffrey Ballet and the chance for the boy to resume a career that the Revolution had done its best to close. At seventeen Juan was entitled to dream, to ignore the odds, and to trust in the inexplicable increase in grace and strength in his maturing body. In joining the Joffrey school he dreamed of stardom and he gave it—more or less—his complete attention.

By 1970 the Joffrey had established a reputation for exciting dance. Adapting classical style to contemporary themes, it aimed—according to Abdullah Jaffa Anver Bey Kahn, otherwise known as Robert Joffrey—to express the boundless release and joy of dancing. To achieve this neo-expressionist goal, it developed a repertoire which, in the words of a New York critic, 'veered from revival of short classics to ballets drenched in media razzmatazz. The company loves to jive, rock, swing, bump and grind. Lights flash, music blares, scenery moves, wind machines blow and both stage and

dancers vibrate and gyrate to electronic devices and music.'
The aim was not to caress, but to blitz the audience.

The assistant director and choreographer was Gerald
Arpino. A trim, compact man with a 'delicate' look, he
added to the enterprise a special preoccupation of his own.
Into the pulsating Joffrey scene he wanted to 'unleash', as
he put it, the American *male* dancer and to establish him
as a star in his own right. But for that to happen, the male
dancer must no longer be considered effeminate; rather, as
one ballet writer put it, he must exhibit 'a virile masculinity,
which is not incompatible with grace and elegance'. How
they tiptoed round the scandal of the homosexual, these
sensitive ballet critics! How they covered their tracks and
dealt in double-talk and cloaked their desires in the high
language of art! At least there was no misunderstanding
Mr Arpino. He was looking for a man, he said, with a torso
like a bull, who would ignite the stage with his potent
sexuality.

In other words, this new male dancer would not be Juan.
With the elegant elongation of his limbs, the slightness of his
lower leg, the delicacy of his head, he was hardly Mr Arpino's
kind of man. That, at least, is the evidence of Juan's folio of
studio photographs, which speak eloquently of his technical
virtuosity. And of his singularity: exceptionally high exten-
sions, a Russian lyricism in the melting, hovering arms and
yet, at the same time, an ethnic tang, a Spanish flourish, a
hint of the matador in the studied bravado of the hand on
the hip and the tilted head. He was exotic, even appealing;
but a far cry from the rampant all-American (white?) male
for whom the choreographer sighed.

Not that Juan was out of sympathy with Mr Arpino's
vision. If the truth be told, he rather sighed for a similar man

himself. And the reason for that, he once told me, lay in the fact that he had a woman's soul in a man's body.

Reflecting on this surprising confession, I wondered if his belief was a fragment of Cuban folk wisdom that he carried secretly within him. Was it, perhaps, a key to self-knowledge that was passed on from one generation of *locas* to another? If this was the case, then you had to concede that the idea had a certain dignity. It meant that a *loca* was neither immoral, nor sick, but simply different.

Yet the doctrine was double-edged. To be an anomaly was in one sense no more remarkable or reprehensible than to be left-handed. It was more disturbing, though, if the woman's soul inside you cried out against the disharmony of her male body and demanded an end to the contradiction. That was how it was with Betty, who submitted herself to the surgeon's knife and happily emerged to resume her business as the proprietress of a hairdressing salon. The other Cubans, including Juan, merely fantasised about such things. In them the woman's soul was never so shrill or insistent, and their male bodies were more assertive. In the gay clubs they amused themselves and teased or appeased their female souls in drag.

La Negra remembered the details. 'We settled into our favourite club,' she told me. 'It was 45th Street and 3rd Avenue, Stage 45, a gigantic disco with a round oak bar. Very chi-chi. Very uppity. I think we were the only poor people there.' They played all sorts of games: La Negra in her accustomed role of *femme fatale*, Alex the ingenue, and Juan/Michel the bimbo, the classic air-head. 'He looked fantastic. He posed—the fashion used to be to pose—looking like a run-way model in his ankle-length fur coat.'

The fur coat was a gift from the priest. Or was it, on

second thoughts, from the engineer, who replaced the priest? Juan was proud of the engineer, the youngest scientist to have worked on the Manhattan Project, he told me, attaching himself to another piece of American history. The engineer must therefore have been a good deal older than the priest, and he was equally bountiful in his affection. If, as we have reason to believe, it is more blessed to give than to receive, Juan provided the occasion for a multiplication of blessings. Nobody could receive more graciously than he, and nobody gave more freely or, I suspect, more patiently, than the engineer. He furnished Juan's apartment like a jewel box with delicate and fashionable things from Bloomingdale's. Years later, when I wrote to him with the news of Juan's death, it was still that mysterious capacity to draw out generosity that he remembered. 'I sense from your account,' he wrote 'that many people are increased in their humanity, more endowed with love, because of Juan's presence among them.'

After the engineer moved to the South to become a distinguished professor there were other men. There was the actor who inflamed him with passion and left him for a woman, which inflamed him still more. And then Ernie, the only one of Juan's patrons whom he dignified with a name, if only because of the indeterminate nature of his business in sporting goods. They each occupied a space in his memory, and he referred to them habitually, and mostly fondly, as if they were a line of popes or kings in whose reign an event could be located. That was the way he ordered his memories, very tidily, in much the same way that he arranged his life, in little compartments, so that there would be no unnecessary confusion or unpleasantness.

But this line of succession was always subordinate to another, more fundamental chronology, an arrangement that turned around the decisive event. Quite simply, there was his life before and his life after the Accident.

It was toward the end of the era of the engineer that the misfortune struck. 'In 1976 my dream ended,' he wrote to the Minister, 'when I was knocked down by a taxi-cab while I was crossing the street to the school of the Joffrey Ballet.' They took him to a city hospital, reconstructed his left knee, and told him he might never walk normally again.

The knee mended. The scar remained, invisibly. He relived the trauma a thousand times. Even ten years later a careless step of mine into the traffic would still set off a panic that always produced a startled-rabbit look in his eyes; he would tense and arch his body and throw back his head, and the surge of anger would last, as he strode off at a furious pace, for several blocks. At every crossroad we were back at the scene of the accident on Sheridan Square.

The dream was ended. Even if he danced again—and in fact the knee recovered more fully than he dared to hope—he would never regain his old strength and fluency. He had foreseen no other future. The accomplishment, the pride in it, that had buoyed him up in the company of Cuban friends was shattered. He was a cot-case, on sickness benefits, then welfare. He was ashamed, turned in on himself, unable to write home.

His memory locked shut around the horror of the next months. For a companion he had Sibley, a black and white cocker spaniel which he alternately spoiled and neglected. Then, after Alex had moved to Los Angeles, he shared his apartment with Rafi, a Puerto Rican dancer whom he loved like a brother. Rafi really was a star. He was a glorious being, with an almost luminous presence. Everybody remembered that. Perhaps that is why the knife that killed him had to be silver. Juan always insisted on this fact. Rafi was murdered, stabbed with the twist of a silver knife in his arse, stabbed and slashed and cut up so badly that you wouldn't want to think about it. 'My best friend,' Juan told the police when they came to ask questions. 'They have killed my best friend in life.'

*

If someone else, some stranger, were telling Juan's story, I expect their chapter might finish here, at the very nadir of his fortunes. That would accord with Juan's own sense of things, and give due weight to the crucial event. And it would restore a fairer balance, some better proportion to the recollection of his life; because already it was more than two-thirds spent.

But this is also my story, and has my memory's shape. And so it continues, relating all those things that happened in New York before we met. Before we began to join our lives.

*

It was a black woman who rescued him from the nightmare. She was, I like to think, like the two black women he knew at the Pink Tea Cup, a homey neighbourhood restaurant in Bleecker Street where they would slap up a plate of Southern fried chicken and collard greens for the cost of no more than a couple of subway rides. Or she was like the more fashionable woman at the Qantas office whom Juan, in later years, would wait to consult about his travel details (there were always problems) even when all the other (white) desks were free. They melted the tension in him, these middle-aged black women, and drew out his boyish sunniness.

32

So at the Welfare office he dealt with a black woman clerk. 'Honey,' she told him one day, 'what's a young man like you doin' on the welfare line? You oughta be ashamed of yourself.' She despatched him forthwith for an audition with an outfit called People Performing Inc. It was a company created out of unemployed artists; it was subsidised by the City and carried out its somewhat chaotic operations in an abandoned building in the East Village.

He went, and his arrival was noticed. Julio, another young unemployed Puerto Rican dancer, saw him come in, clutching his folio of studio photographs. He was wearing a cream silk shirt, brown boots and khaki pants with the kind of knife-edge crease that pleased his Cuban sense of being well groomed. As the only other Latin in this odd assemblage of crazies and supposed artists, Juan gravitated to Julio in an instant alliance. Playing on Julio's well-founded reservations about the enterprise, he put on an act of campy outrage that achieved its comic effect from his own obvious vulnerability. 'How dare Welfare send me to this place! None of these people', he told Julio, 'have my experience.'

Experienced or not, they had a show to put on. It was nearly Christmas—a festival that Juan regarded distantly as a kind of ethnic celebration for WASPs—and they had been commissioned to produce the City's annual tribute to 'A Visit from St Nicholas'. Directing this quaint piece of family entertainment was a gentleman who, according to the programme notes, was otherwise preoccupied with a biographical montage of movement, text and sound on the life of Jean Genet. The technical designer was an astrologer; an expressionist painter with a passion for metaphysics prepared the sets; and the music was provided variously by a cow-bell artiste, a guitarist who danced at the Continental

Baths and a 'red-hot, white-skin blues artist' called Leatherman.

Though he knew there were no long-term prospects in this quixotic company of counter-cultural relics, Juan was back on his feet. He began to reinvent a future: a dance workshop, perhaps, for Spanish kids on the Lower East Side; teaching; choreography. In dance you have to prepare for getting older. Then Julio discovered an interesting possibility, and six months later Juan followed him. He became a scholarship student in the dance programme at Marymount Manhattan College.

Marymount had begun its prestigious history as a finishing school for young Catholic ladies. Here their manners and their morals were polished and refined until, having acquired all the graces that society and matrimony would require of them, they graduated in a flurry of brocade and white lace. On these ceremonial occasions they received their certificates of virtue from the Cardinal Archbishop who, to judge from the pictures, had the habit of regularly upstaging his daughters in sartorial splendour. The evidence of their progress, class by class and year by year—and of his magnificence—was framed and mounted in sequence on the wall of the college library. Juan puzzled over this display. Were these his sisters, part of the pedigree that he could claim? Or were they tormentors, perpetrating some white respectable female joke on a Hispanic queen of no particular virtue? The questions remained unresolved.

By the time that they threw open their doors to men and established a scholarship programme, the Marymount sisters had long since embraced the values of progressive education. But their institute retained its aura of privilege. In the morning before classes began, sleek limousines continued to deliver long-faced, long-haired and long-limbed young ladies to the door of the neo-Georgian facade in the most elegant section of East 71st Street.

Although it didn't yet boast a male changing room for the dance students, you would have to say, as Juan frequently did, that Marymount had class. For many of the students this seemed so self-evident and so appropriate that it went unremarked. For Juan, on the other hand, it required a sharp alertness and a certain inventiveness. If they returned from their summer vacations in Paris or skiing holidays in Switzerland, he would regale them with stories of Brazil, or the Caribbean, where an unexplained profusion of cousins was constantly inviting him. Otherwise he wrapped himself in an air of privacy, a mode of existence that can also be interpreted as classy in New York. Only the cook knew that he slipped into the kitchen of the college canteen after the lunch hour for a free feed.

The coursework posed other problems. Dance classes he approached nonchalantly, even with a touch of arrogance. The academic classes excited him more, but they also distressed him. In one routine exercise he was required to write a critique of a ballet he had recently seen; but if he was stringing together a tenuous existence on scholarships and grants, and falling behind with his rent, and jumping the subway turnstiles because he didn't have the money for a token, he was unlikely to be swanning about with the critical public at the ballet.

That was the least of his problems with this exercise. From his Cuban education he retained the ability to recite the patriotic poems of José Martí. He could count to a hundred in Russian. And he had more recently acquired a High School Equivalency Diploma to which the Regents of the

University of the State of New York had affixed their seal; but none of this conferred on him the important ability to write. Despite this disadvantage, he submitted a piece describing a Joffrey performance of Gerald Arpino's 'Trinity'. It began with panache. 'Sneers, leers and cutting remarks have almost become the traditional property of the balletomanes and their adamant opponents, the devotees of the modern dance.' It came back with a scribbled comment in lipstick pink. 'Is this your wording? No credit.'

The next semester a longer piece on Diaghilev met the same fate. 'As a personal choice,' this essay concluded, 'if only one of Diaghilev's ballets could be saved for the future, I would choose Apollo, for its pure beauty and expressive use of style.' The professor pounced. 'It is one thing to take material directly from a book; another to give it as a personal opinion!' The logic of the professor was impeccable; these were obviously different 'things'. Yet if one's personal opinion should in fact happen to coincide with that of another author, it is difficult to see why this pleasing coincidence should be judged more harshly than the act of plagiarism itself.

Being a liberal college, they gave him another chance, and then another. Naturally it was not the task of a dance professor to explain to him the rules of English grammar or the construction of English sentences, or how an essay might be shaped or argued. And so, equally naturally, the dispiriting succession of savaged essays continued.

There was more joy for him in the college theatre. He sewed costumes, painted make-up, and danced. In his last semester the students presented a programme of modern dance. 'Motion Madness', as they called it, was a flamboyant show-biz extravaganza, belted out to the strains of Bill Haley and Dr Buzzard's Original Savannah Band. Strangely, the production was prefaced by a piece called 'Expressions', a *pas de deux* to Debussy's 'Reverie' of such porcelain delicacy that it might have been choreographed for some defunct European court. This was the work—though the middle initial made him sound more like a banker than an artist—of Juan G. Céspedes.

Of course it was a great show. That was affirmed again and again as the audience dissolved in a welter of congratulations to their performing daughters. Well-heeled Hispanic ladies with red fingernails lowered their *hauteur* in the excitement; Westchester matrons, with that severely anorexic look that rich American women are apt to confuse with elegance, allowed their modest bosoms to swell with pride.

I was in the audience that night. Sitting with me, making use of the other free passes to which the performers were entitled, were Hiram and Danny. Hiram was none other than La Negra. He had preceded Juan to New York, where he had settled into a small apartment in the Village and a relationship with Danny. In New York he had discovered his Jewish roots, though Juan maintained in private that if his family in Cuba had any religion, at best they were Seventh Day Adventists, which, in Juan's normally tolerant opinion, was hardly a religion at all. Nevertheless, there was no doubt that Hiram was deeply observant. He always lit the Sabbath candles and said the prayers, which more than compensated for the occasional cigarette he allowed himself on Saturday afternoons. He also attached great importance to the tradition of not cutting one's hair. This observance he also laid on Danny, who was otherwise more at home in leather than a tallis but who, for the sake of domestic harmony, had grown his greying hair thick and long and plaited in a pig-tail. That is why, as I sat beside him in the auditorium, he reminded me more of a Chinese mandarin than the traditional Jew Hiram apparently intended him to be.

They—or perhaps I should now say we—were Juan's family. In company he generally introduced Hiram as his cousin, which adequately reflected the bond that had developed between them. He was Juan's essential link with Guantánamo, his source of news during all the months when he never bothered to write. In Hiram's apartment they laughed and watched TV and ate *caramelo* and smoked and argued together. If Juan sometimes bridled at Hiram's superior airs or doubted his claims to be psychic, Hiram retaliated by accusing him of being secretive or, if he really wanted to hurt, by hinting that Juan had not made it. Betty was doing well in her hairdressing salon; it seemed that Alex had fallen on his feet in Los Angeles: and Hiram himself, despite the ulcer that he nursed, was happily settled with the ever-reliable Danny.

As for Juan, at the age of twenty-seven he was still a college student. He clung to that, but he was on shaky ground, making slow progress, and Marymount, which had already reduced his grant, was soon to close its doors on him as a failure. In 1980 the apartment he had maintained for the best part of ten years was sold, or he fell behind with his rent, depending on whose story one believes. Either way, the result was the same. He was evicted. Sibley the cocker spaniel was given away. He packed his household goods and his fur into a couple of tea-chests and stored them in a warehouse on the other side of the Brooklyn Bridge for fifty dollars a month. He bundled his clothes into a carry-bag and left it in a locker at the Port Authority Bus Terminal. He was on the street.

CHAPTER THREE

A prodigal summer, though the gardens dried.
Burdened with so much happiness,
I knew the web of joy must sometime tear.

—Barbara Giles, 'Cobweb Summer'

On Friday 3 July 1981 I went to early Mass. By the end of the Mass the priest was sweating. Summertime in New York, I was discovering, was drenched with sweat, though it was rarely so pure an essence as the kind that impregnated the wafer I received from the priest's damp hand. On the subway, sweat sickly mingled with cheap scent; in the gay bars on Christopher Street it hit you in a mixture of amyl or diffused in the acrid drift of marijuana smoke; on the streets it came at you out of peripatetic hot-dog stands or the open doors of greasy-spoon cafes.

Walking home from church, with my shirt already wet on my back, I bought a copy of the *Times* and turned in at Nick the Greek's for my usual eggs and coffee. On the eve of a holiday weekend it was less than normally busy. There was room at a corner table to spread out the paper, a small but significant luxury which disposed me cheerfully to the day ahead. There was no news of any moment, which may explain why I spent so long reading the almost full-page advertisement of the Independence Savings Bank. 'Sing out on the Fourth!' it said, and to encourage this holiday spirit it printed the music and three verses of the 'Star Spangled Banner':

What is that which the breeze, o'er the towering steep,
As it fitfully blows half conceals, half discloses?

So much glory is hard to take at breakfast and so the *Times*, which is a newspaper of impeccable taste, balanced this rich fare with a thin column of more astringent medical reporting. Doctors in California and New York had diagnosed among homosexual men forty-one cases of a rare and often rapidly fatal form of cancer. The cancer appeared in violet-coloured spots which might be taken for bruises and which often turned brown before they spread through the body. Eight victims had already died, but other cases might have gone undetected because of the rarity of the condition and the difficulty even dermatologists might have in diagnosing it. It seemed to have something to do with promiscuous sex. Most of the cases had involved homosexual men who had had multiple and frequent sexual encounters each night up to four times a week.

By the time I had arrived at the bottom of the column I felt reassured. The *Times* made it sound like an exercise in mental arithmetic. If x men have sex y times a night and on z nights each week, calculate the number of encounters that will take place in New York in a year. This was definitely not serious. Or at least, it did not concern me. I was not in the violet-spot league.

Three weeks later I met Juan. That was not very serious either, a chance encounter, much like any other, except that it was on 14th Street by the steps of Our Lady of Guadaloupe's chapel. I was on my way to the Public Library; he was on his way home, as he put it, from a disco. He was going out to sleep on the sofa of a friend in New Jersey. When we spoke, he took me to be English which, on his carefully calibrated scale of sophistication, was better than average, though he would have preferred me to be French. He established that I was, as he called it, a professor of history, though he found it odd that I had no printed card to corroborate the fact. Where did I live? 'On Eighth Avenue, just around the corner.' We had reached the point in this ritual exchange of detail where someone had to make a move. Suddenly he reached out his arm and squeezed the left nipple through my blackwatch tartan shirt. 'Let's go to your place,' he said. So we did, and after we had had sex he fell asleep and slept till late in the afternoon, when he woke up and said, 'I'm hungry.'

It happened that 25 July, the day which we always kept as our anniversary, was the Feast of St James. To celebrate the occasion, our undistinguished stretch of 14th Street between Seventh and Eighth Avenues, before it crosses into no-man's land towards the river, was holding a party. More salubrious neighbourhoods in the heart of the Village timed their street parties for the autumn, and they sold mixed-grain breads and gourmet salads and herbal oils decanted into little stoppered bottles. But 14th Street is Spanish, and in the evening, when we reappeared, it was filled with the aroma of roasting pork, and there were stands selling *tamales* and convivial groups drinking beer at the pavement tables outside the cafes. We lingered over a meal for which, in an unspoken agreement, I picked up the bill. And when the dancing was becoming ragged and the coals on the charcoal grills were dying, and it was nearly midnight, we went home again, and he never left.

Michel. He was called Michel. An unexpected name, I thought, for a Cuban. I was uncomfortable with it. It might have sounded fine in Paris but here, well, it struck me as unconvincing, stagey and—quite frankly—too transparently camp. Of course in America you never ceased to be surprised by names. My own landlord had been christened Gaylord, which had not prevented him from having a discreet and mildly successful career in the State Department. And it was true that, with use, even a name like that could begin to take on the sober and serious characteristics of the person to whom it was attached. But Michel? I resisted it.

It was several days before I learned that he had another name. He was sitting at my desk, filling out a college application form.

'Juan Gualberto?'

'Yes,' he said, 'it's my official name.'

He thought it was common, and no doubt in Cuba it was. Yet I liked the way it sounded, full-bodied and rich like red wine.

'I'd like to call you Juan,' I said.

He shrugged. 'With my friends I am Michel,' he countered. Still, if that was what I preferred, he wouldn't object. It was no big deal.

There comes a moment in a casual encounter when the energy in which it was conceived exhausts itself; the small talk dries up, and by mutual consent the meeting is deemed to be without significance. To my surprise the conversation with Juan continued to flow, to eddy with unexpected surges and to relapse into comfortable silences. I liked the manner of his speaking, the richly eccentric idiom, the unpredictable syntax, the smattering of Spanish curses. When he reproached me with not listening, as occasionally he did, he underestimated the pleasure that his voice alone could give.

Without ever having decided to do so, we were living together. It was a convenient arrangement. He had no home; I was alone; and in his company the city seemed to acquire a fresh charm, as though August had turned into magical May. He knew the streets like the back of his hand, and together we roamed spaciously through Soho and Chinatown and the East Village. He knew cheap places to eat, and introduced me to the women at the Pink Tea Cup and then to the cook at Chino's, a dowdy little Chinese Cuban cafe with a decor, if you could call it that, so authentically fifties that it was in danger of becoming chic. He was upset to hear that I had been mugged on my second day in New York, though he considered I had been inexcusably careless and volunteered himself as a survival guide. I had to get street-smart.

'But that was months ago!' I protested.

'No matter,' he said, 'don't dawdle; avoid eye-contact.'

'But what if I hadn't looked at you?'

'Well,' he said, 'with faggots it's different.' His concern touched me, and I was attracted to a strange sense of innocence in him, though of what he was innocent I could never quite decide.

As we began to unpack our pasts, he was curious to hear about my travels. I had been to India. Why would I go there, he wanted to know. Wasn't it full of hippies and crazy gurus and miserable poverty? No, he disapproved of India; they had no right to spend all that money on nuclear weapons when the people were living in poverty. But when he heard that I had spent some time in Israel, he was all attention.

I told him about Jerusalem and how its walls were golden in the light of the morning sun and white in the light of the moon; how I had walked in a procession of palms that came down from the Mount of Olives and made its way through St Stephen's gate to the courtyard of St Anne; and how the Arab boys sat on the walls on either side of the entrance to the city, swinging their legs and waving to their friends in the procession. He was interested in the Arab boys. 'Do they make out?' he wanted to know. I supposed that they did.

Sometimes, if I asked him, he would talk about Cuba. He told me the story of his escape, and of his dismissal from the Ballet School, and of the one time he had seen Fidel and cheered for him along with the rest of the crowd. And he talked about the Yoruba, his people, who had come across the sea in chains from Nigeria, bringing their religion with them, the religion of Changó and Obatalá, the white creator of the world, and Babalú Ayé, the god of illness.

'But I thought Cuba was a Catholic country?'

'Well, yes,' he said, 'we are Catholics. But there it's different. We have St Bárbara and Lázaro and the Virgen de la Caridad.'

'But don't you have them here?'

My questions exasperated him. 'Johnny,' he said, 'you don't understand.'

In my ignorance I had no idea that we were verging on the subject of *santería*, that fusion of African and Catholic belief that pervades the religious imagination of Cuba. Whenever we came close to this mystery he shied away, embarrassed by this evidence of Third World primitivism, or shy of my intolerance, unable or unwilling to say how the gods may be propitiated by the sacrifice of cocks and pigeons, how they may enter the body of initiates, and how they may be worshipped in a trance to the beating of sacred drums. I let the matter drop.

Sometimes the balance of our conversations was reversed, and it was he who asked the questions for which I had no answer. Like, 'Why did Hitler hate the Jews?' That question arose when I was telling him about the research that had brought me to New York. I was working on the history of a dynasty of German-Jewish industrialists, a classic tale of rags to riches acted out over three generations. In the last generation, before the Nazis brutally intervened and 'Aryanised' the firm, the three heirs to the family fortune were already well on the way to squandering their inheritance. Clara's husband invested her share in a bank which crashed in the depression; Klaus led a drifting existence on the fringes of the Weimar literary scene; and Hans, who managed the firm, was more preoccupied with society life in Berlin than with the industrial realities of the provincial town on which the family fortunes depended. After each day at the archive I recounted the next episode, the latest detail, in the saga of the family's gathering disaster, and Juan was always ready for more. For Klaus in particular he had a soft spot. He was impressed when I discovered that in 1933 Klaus had acted as a secret courier for Thomas Mann in Switzerland; he was delighted when I was able to report that Klaus had escaped the Nazis and joined the Foreign Legion; and he was puzzled to learn that he finally saw out the war in hiding as a gardener to a Vichy comtesse. What was the nature of the relationship? we wondered. I inclined to a Lady Chatterley solution. Juan, on the other hand, had long since formed the opinion that Klaus was gay.

This mystery prompted him to drop in at the archive one afternoon. If he could see a photograph of Klaus, he was sure he would be able to establish his sexual identity. Surprised by this unannounced visit, this sudden escape of our private life into the workplace, I came downstairs from the reading room to find him in sympathetic conversation —which is to say that he was politely listening—with the receptionist. She was a lady of advanced middle age, and as she had also to attend to membership subscriptions and the regular mailing lists, it was generally if uncharitably supposed in the Institute that the repetitive nature of her job had imprinted itself on the operation of her mental processes. I arrived in the lobby in time to catch the end of the story of her Uncle Karl who had been an officer in the *Luftwaffe*, so it was strange, wasn't it, she said to Juan, that she was working in a Jewish institute? He agreed that indeed it was, which pleased her, and we went upstairs past the portraits of the German-Jewish Nobel prizewinners to inspect the photos.

He became a regular visitor to the Institute, and the receptionist was always pleased to see him. 'That nice young man is here to see you,' she would say to me over the internal phone. Although he never acquired the distinction of a name, she accepted him into the routine of her day as unquestioningly as she aired each of the nine rooms in her apartment for precisely five minutes each morning. It was not for her to comment on the dynamics of a cross-colour, cross-class, same-sex relationship that had materialised in her lobby.

In this respect the bishop was less reticent, and certainly more knowing. I am not in the habit of entertaining bishops, but when they cross your path there is no reason why they should not be shown the same consideration as lesser mortals. This prelate was a friend of a common friend; and as he happened to be passing through Manhattan and had no pressing ecclesiastical business on a Saturday afternoon, he invited himself to tea. It was rumoured that he had left his island diocese under a cloud, and whether it was this hint of scandal, or simply the grandeur of the occasion (which would greatly impress Hiram in the re-telling) that attracted Juan, I cannot say; but he determined to overcome his shyness and stay in to meet the bishop.

In his usual unhurried way he was still in the shower when the doorbell rang. There was therefore no opportunity to effect the usual introductions. The bishop settled into our single armchair and proceeded to relate to me the latest theological enterprise on which he had embarked. He was writing a work on the spirituality of sex or—given his celibate condition—perhaps it was a study of the sexuality of the spirit. In any event, it was a subject much under-investigated by religious writers. At this point, the bathroom door opened, and in a billow of steam and a cloud of aftershave and a hint of some more elusive fragrance that he had probably picked up from a demonstration in Bloomingdale's cosmetic department, Juan made his entrance. 'This', I said to the bishop, 'is Juan,' which seemed the very least I could offer by way of explanation. They exchanged brief pleasantries, and then, when he had satisfied himself that it was a real bishop with an amethyst ring, Juan was gone, looking more youthful than ever.

'How old is that child?' the bishop enquired.

'Twenty-seven,' I replied, and supposed from the arching of his eyebrows that I stood doubly convicted, not only of pederasty but untruthfulness as well!

In fact, though not in the way that the bishop implied, it was difficult to know what the truth of our situation was. I had never imagined a relationship like this. I did not see myself in the role of the priest or the engineer. Nor did I feel any special affinity with Christopher Isherwood chasing his working-class boys in Berlin, or with E. M. Forster doting on his Alexandrian tram conductor. On the contrary, I brooded over the disparity in our backgrounds and the divergence of our interests, to say nothing of the fact that our homes—that word again—were half a world apart. When I thought about it rationally, I could not avoid the conclusion that there was no future in this. It was no more than a summer fling, not so much an affair as a diversion in place of the holiday that I couldn't afford to take out of town. The summer had thrown us together, and now that the August days were at an end, it was time to part. Fond of him as I was, he was not the lover I was obscurely looking for. Nor, I was sure, did I measure up to the man of his dreams, a rich man with a house and a car who would give him a diamond ring and keep him in ease. In fairness to us both—that is how I put it to myself—I should ask him to go.

That was my mood—or rather one of my moods—on the last day of summer. 'I am fitfully devising a strategy of withdrawal,' I wrote to my friend Rickard, who was holed up in the English countryside at a place called Rabbit Hill, where there was nothing to do but write.

I did ask him to leave. It was late in the afternoon when I broached the subject. He was sitting on the bed, cross-legged, sewing buttons on a shirt. Coolly, as objectively as I could manage, I said that I had been thinking. About us. And about where we were heading. And that, well, there wasn't really room for two people in this tiny studio apartment. I felt cramped.

Then, sensing what was coming, he counter-attacked on an unexpected flank. 'What about that fat woman from the church? She takes up space. She's been here twice this week. What does she want?'

'She only wants to talk.'

He didn't believe me. 'She's disgusting. I don't want you to bring her here.'

He was sitting upright now, growing tense, preparing to defend himself.

'She needs a good shampoo,' he said.

It suddenly dawned on me that, incredibly, he was jealous, that he saw a competitor in this woman who wanted only to discuss theology and join the South American missions.

'Well, this is ridiculous,' I replied, 'I mean, whose apartment is this? You can't just invite yourself into someone's apartment and take it over as if you intend to stay for ever.'

'I didn't invite myself. We came together.'

That was stretching a point, though it was at least as close to the truth as my version of events.

'I don't care how we came here. What I'm trying to say is that there isn't room for both of us. I can't live like this.'

'So where do you want me to go?'

That was the question I had been dreading. I said nothing and let the storm that I had stirred up break over me.

'I'm not going,' he yelled. 'For ten years I had an apartment and they threw me on the street. Ten years! *Carajo!* Johnny! Do you hear what I'm telling you? I'm not going.'

He was working himself into a frenzy. He hurled his sewing kit across the room. Tears sprang in his eyes and then, no longer able to contain his wild emotion, he stormed out and slammed the door behind him.

Well after midnight when the doorbell rang, I got up to let him in. We didn't speak. He poked about in the fridge looking for something to eat. And then, when he slipped into bed, I knew, despite myself, I was glad that he was back.

Three weeks later, in my next letter to Rickard, there was the merest echo of our row, and of my capitulation:

At any moment [I wrote], I'm expecting the phone to ring. At the other end will be my Cuban friend who, in typical New York style, will be ringing to let me know he is about to knock on the door. [Had I still not given him a key?] This odd custom supposedly prevents you getting mugged and at the same time handsomely increases the profits of the telephone company.

To my great surprise, and despite my frequent fits of wanting to be alone, etc., we are still together. He is patient, persistent and generally nice, and infuriates me—unreasonably—by always reading first any bits of news in the paper about astronauts, missiles and anything else that might be happening in space. I am crotchety, querulous and crabby, but my blue eyes apparently compensate for these defects. Not that I'm even convinced that my eyes *are* blue; but they are close enough, especially in a city like this where brown eyes must preponderate by a ratio of 90 to 10. Anyway, it's all very innocent and comfortable for the time being.

Patience was not normally a quality I associated with Juan. The explanation of it here was simple. One night between the August and September letters he had confided, half-apologetically, 'I'm sorry, Johnny, but I think I'm falling a little bit in love.' I ignored it as best I could. Being a little bit in love was not much different, I hoped, from being a little drunk. It would pass. It would have to, because I was planning to move on to Germany for the next stage of my research on Hans and Klaus. 'Although I have the best part of four months left in N.Y.C.,' my letter to Rickard concluded, 'I'm beginning to get a kind of itchy-feet end-of-my-stay feeling, which manifests itself in more frequent recourse to the Xerox machine.' I would soon need to renew my passport but would delay it as long as possible because the cost had gone up to $35. Money was tight. 'What a mean note for the end of a letter,' I concluded. There was a PS. 'The phone rang!'

For the next few weeks we bracketed out the uncertain future. But already, I remember, Cuba was beginning to permeate our life together with its tastes and moods and extravagances. It appeared in the supermarket trolley in the form of *adobo*, a spicy mixture of herbs intended to relieve the blandness of my cooking. It came home in the shape of green bananas which, I was informed, were *plátanos* and which had to be fried and pounded into a flat cake and fried again and sprinkled with salt in precisely the way that Clara de la Rosa had done in the kitchen at Guantánamo. Cuba also dictated that we observe the ritual of a Saturday-night investment in the lottery, and at other times as well if there happened to be a couple of spare dollars in the jar on the mantelpiece. And of course this was perfectly reasonable. Juan had already formed a realistic estimate of the modest income of a junior academic, and how else, he asked me, could we hope to be rich? In his view, riches and success, fame and fortune were largely a matter of luck, and this being the case it was foolish to deny oneself the chance of being lucky. The lottery became an obligation. Failing to buy a ticket was not simply (wilful) forgetfulness on my part; it was moral delinquency.

In the autumn the pace of the city quickened. The college semester began at Marymount and Juan was immersed in preparing his Debussy-inspired ballet. He rehearsed in the evenings, and I found myself waiting for him to come home, making dinner at midnight, anxious to hear the details of his progress, and as nervous as he was as the day of the show approached. Sometimes, if he was not home too late, we would light the fire and toast marshmallows and drink red wine from the liquor store across the road. The unaccustomed wine made him drowsy, and more often than not, he would fall asleep with his head on my lap. Then, gazing into the fire, I would revert, obsessively, to the undecided matter of our future.

So often had I circled round this question that I knew by now every move my mind would make, and every counter-move. The more my rational self declared against the prospect of a life together, the more strongly I desired it. And at the back of my mind, whenever I pitched up at this impasse, there flickered the memory of a conversation that had taken place in Melbourne some months before. 'The trouble with you,' I had been told by a friend, the way only a friend would say, 'The trouble with you is that you won't commit yourself. You won't let yourself be loved.' It had been an after-dinner observation and, as such, I could have easily dismissed it. Instead, though without allowing there was any substance to it, I had pressed him to explain his opinion. Why should I refuse what I most wanted? 'I think you're afraid of getting hurt,' he said. Well, perhaps I was; and perhaps there was nothing unusual in that. But how could I tell if what he said were true? Whenever I tried to measure his words against my knowledge of myself, I became confused, and other voices that were in me, other memories, resisted any clear admission of his claim. I was back at the impasse. Only one thing was clear about Juan and me. Here he was, here we were; and we were happy.

In that autumn semester he also enrolled in a video class. Each student in turn was entrusted with the video equipment for a weekend, and the assignment was to film a happening in the city. When Juan's turn came, we looked in the 'What's On' column in the *Village Voice* and discovered that there was, remarkably, nothing much listed except a housing demonstration in Hell's Kitchen. Compared with Juan's TV-induced fantasy of filming Diana Ross in concert in Central Park with a cast of thousands, the People's Coalition for Better Housing was hardly glamorous. He was reluctant to revisit the scene of his own first days in New York; he was apprehensive about his ability to handle the equipment; and he was, justifiably, even more nervous about having enlisted me as his technical assistant.

After a considerable hike from the subway station, we arrived at the demonstration outside a tenement block that reeked of boiled cabbage and tom-cat. There were speeches denouncing Reagan and the city administration and the developers, and then the demonstration formed itself into a motley procession that moved off around the corner of Ninth Avenue, where a black revival meeting was in full cry. At this point Juan discovered that I had bungled the sound recording, which I now belatedly switched on when he was expostulating loudly over the hubbub of the Gospel choir. When this piece of *cinema vérité* was duly exhibited in class at Marymount, the first sound to be heard was an agitated Spanish-American voice shouting furiously: '*Carajo*, Johnny. I told you to turn on the fucking sound!' He got a D for technique which we both agreed was my fault, but the grade

53

was redeemed to C+ because, the professor told him, of his social compassion.

I have one other memory of that November afternoon: the wind. It whipped off the river sharp and mean, and we were glad to step down from the street into the musty warmth of the subway on our way home. Juan was still living out of the bag of summer clothes that he had deposited, and since retrieved, at the Port Authority Bus Terminal. His winter jackets and coat, together with the other things he had saved from the apartment, were still in storage at the warehouse. He had already fallen two months behind with the extortionate rental payments, and until those payments were made they refused him access to his locker. So there was nothing for it but to part with the money, which I did ungraciously, and the prize specimen of Brooklyn manhood in the warehouse office returned the compliment and flicked the key at us with venomous contempt.

We located the locker on the third floor at the end of a long corridor; we heard a dog barking; and there was a flickering fluorescent light that might have been designed to emphasise the overwhelming desolation of this place.

Juan pulled out the two tea-chests. They had both been ransacked. The stereo was gone. The portable TV was gone. A few bits of crockery were smashed. Digging deeper into the muddle of pullovers and jackets, he pulled out two plaster statues, the kind I had seen in *botánicas*, religious knick-knack shops that sell holy oils and curative herbs and magical candles. The statues had lost their heads. 'Bárbara and Lázaro,' he said, and I could see that he was going to cry. He sat down on the concrete floor with the meagre trophies of his twelve years in America strewn about him.

Miraculously the fur coat was still there, and I gathered it up and wrapped it round his shoulders.

I can't remember exactly when I said that I loved him, but it could have been there in the warehouse, on the far side of the Brooklyn Bridge.

CHAPTER FOUR

When the German passport official asked him the purpose of his journey, he could have truthfully replied, 'I'm looking for my homeland and I've come to find out if this is it.'

—Christopher Isherwood, *Christopher and His Kind*

At the end of February I left for Berlin to continue my work on Hans, Klaus and their family in the German archives. It was a subdued farewell at JFK. When I passed through the departure gate, I knew that he would be heading back into the city with nowhere to go. We had made a couple of efforts to find him an apartment—a room with barred windows on 168th Street and another place at the end of the A-line in Jamaica—but anywhere remotely affordable was so depressing or so dangerous that we gave up in despair. He had enough money for a few nights at the 'Y', and after that he would wear out his welcome on the sofa of one friend after another.

'Don't worry about me, Johnny,' he said. He would get by.

We had firmly agreed that as soon as the semester was over he would come to spend the summer with me in Berlin. He wanted to believe in this arrangement, but I doubt that he did. If there was anything in New York more familiar than a shattered dream, it was a broken promise. 'I'll call you,' they said. 'We'll be in touch.' The usual courtesies of the transient lover already on the lookout for a new adventure, no more than a civilised parting ritual, with not too much fuss. Although he preferred a little more drama in his own disengagements, this, he knew, was the way things end.

When the cheque for his airline ticket finally arrived, he was elated, 'like a cat with a dish of cream', Hiram told me, and I wished I could have seen him like that. His stocks rose in the circle of his Cuban friends, who conceded that there appeared to be something serious in this affair after all. But the cheque was the least of our problems. Transferring money from one country to another is considerably easier than transferring persons, particularly a person like Juan.

At the beginning of June I intended to be in London to do some business on behalf of the University Library. I suggested to Juan that he buy a return ticket to London and, after a couple of days there, we could travel back together by train to Berlin. This suggestion did not meet with his approval. Paris was still the destination of his dreams. He combed New York searching for a ticket that would take him there, and finally came up with a cheap student flight that would land him in Amsterdam and, at the end of the summer, fly him out on a specified date from Paris. This, he was sure, was value for money; with train trips to London and Berlin, he would stop over in four countries compared with my plan for two.

Despite these changes, we still planned to meet in London. I was at Victoria Station early on the appointed evening, waiting for the boat train to deliver him from Amsterdam. He was also early, but waiting in mounting anxiety at the Victoria Coach Station, where he had been deposited after a flight to Gatwick. By the time he had discovered the mistake and made his way to the railway station in the care of a London bobby, he was almost hysterical. He was tired, hungry and unforgiving, and his disposition was not improved by a meal in the nearest Wimpy Bar. At the bed-and-breakfast place where we stayed, nylon sheets and soggy toast added to his determined unhappiness. He was impossible; and although I had grown accustomed to his *penchant* for melodrama, which might have been appropriate to the misunderstanding at Victoria, I was puzzled and distressed at the persistence of his hostile irritability.

In mid-morning, as I was trying to prise him out of the bedroom, the Life Guard obligingly marched past our window on their way to the Palace. The sheer surprise lifted him out of his surliness and, seizing the moment, we traipsed after the Guard to watch them perform their ceremonial change. With his face pressed against the railings of Buckingham Palace, he hoped that the Queen would appear; and when she did, he would tell her what he thought of her country and her soggy toast and bitter marmalade, though he would have to admit that she had turned on a very good show with the royal wedding twelve months earlier, and he thoroughly approved the way she had put that pert little Nancy Reagan in her place.

This conversation with the Queen appeared to relax him, and as we walked away down the Mall he began to explain the problem. Americans, as we knew, did not need a visa to travel in Western Europe. But Juan, as I now recalled, was not an American citizen. It was only by chance that he had learned, on the day before he left New York, that he would need a visa for each country he visited. In the last twenty-four hours he had secured an entry permit for Holland and the UK, but for Germany he had no permit.

We examined his passport. It turned out not to be a passport at all, but simply a permit to re-enter the United States. But in case the possession of this document should give him a false sense of security, or any illusion concerning his place in the world, there was a notice inside that said he shouldn't take it for granted that they would let him back in.

> Persons who have been convicted of or admit having committed a felony or other crime or misdemeanour involving moral turpitude either before or after entering the United States, other criminal, immoral, insane, mentally or physically defective aliens, those afflicted with loathsome or contagious diseases, are subject to exclusion if attempting to re-enter, notwithstanding they may be in possession of permits to re-enter.

Compared with my own passport, which pompously requested various foreign personages to let me pass without let or hindrance on pain of the Governor-General's displeasure, this miserable document almost gloated at the possibility of disowning him. He was a stateless person. In a gentler world this condition would have much to recommend it; in the actual world of policed immigration and passport controls, it was at best humiliating and at worst potentially disastrous.

The next morning we presented ourselves at the German Consulate to apply for the necessary permit. I entered the building first, through a revolving glass door that was guarded on the inside by a couple of terrorist-repellent security men. Juan followed, but when he stepped inside, they body-searched him. Standing beside him in the queue,

I could sense him bristle. They were racists, these Germans. Why had they not frisked me? He was right, of course, and I knew it. I tried to pacify him, to brush the incident aside. We had come to get a visa, and there was nothing to be gained by launching the civil rights movement all over again in a German consular office in London.

The next man through the door was an African, and he too was searched. And so was an Arab-looking gentleman. Then came a European, a white middle-aged business type to whom the guards nodded deferentially as he took his place in the line. Juan exploded.

'Search that man!' he shouted with such electrifying effect that you would think a gun-toting terrorist had stormed into the lobby. 'Why don't you search that man?' he screamed, jabbing a finger at the businessman who, to my relief, was immediately whisked away to another section to complete his privileged arrangements undisturbed.

We reached the counter.

'How long do you want?' asked the clerk.

'Two months.'

'I'm sorry. With this document only two weeks are permitted. Come back in four weeks to collect it.'

We were stunned. Anticipating a short stay in London, I had brought only a small amount of money with me, and Juan, as usual, had virtually none. We couldn't tell that to the clerk.

'Does it normally take four weeks to issue a visa?' I enquired.

'With that document, yes,' he replied, glaring at Juan as though he were looking for signs of a loathsome disease. 'He should have applied in New York.'

'But we didn't know.'

The official shrugged. That was all. 'Next.'

Outside on the footpath we argued.

'You betrayed me, Johnny!'

'What do you mean?'

'You know what I mean. You sided with those whiteys.'

It was the first time that colour had ever come between us. Bridling at this accusation and unwilling to acknowledge any guilt, I repeated my line that there was no point in creating a scene if we wanted to get the visa. With a twist of the knife he replied, 'And did we get the visa?'

He was being bloody-minded, I told myself. Why should he punish me because of this chance affront? Or, if I conceded that it was not *mere* chance, how did he expect me to take on the whole colossus of prejudice that this little scene encapsulated?

'That's just what you would say,' I could hear him reply. 'You're always so cool, so logical, so sure you can work the system. So white! It wasn't you they treated like a criminal. You didn't feel a rage so deep inside you that it ran all over your body and made you tremble and scream and look like a madman. No, you just let them do it.'

I was a whitey. And this England, he reminded me, was my ancestral home. These were my people. When I looked around at those South Kensington faces, freshly flushed with pride at their Falklands victory, I felt no kinship with them. In New York it had not been like this. Only London made me feel really foreign. London, and Juan.

At a pinch I had enough money to last a week in London. There seemed no alternative but to leave Juan in England, return to Berlin alone and attempt to pull some strings from the German end to expedite the visa. But where was he to stay in the meantime? One option was Lincoln, where my friends the Gribbens were ensconced with their children, Christopher and Rosie, in a picture postcard Georgian house. From the front window of the house you looked out directly on to the great west facade of the cathedral. Juan refused to be impressed. He didn't give a damn about carved choir-stalls or floriated finials or the Lincoln Imp. And the wintry weather of that June, the chill of the Georgian house and the positively arctic temperature in the massive church depressed him still further.

'If this is Europe,' he said, 'forget it. Forget it. I'm going home.'

I half wished he would. And in the very act of contemplating that impossibility, for I knew they would never alter the return date of his charter-flight ticket, I was ashamed and fearful of my treachery. I wanted to say, 'Don't push me. Don't push me any further.' Yet I could hardly trust myself to speak at all. I was exasperated by his rudeness, almost beyond endurance. I was hurt by the way he rebuffed me. I felt crushed by the burden of his dependence, and I resented his resentment. If he felt trapped in this unlikely city on a hill, so far from the Europe of his imagining, then so did I: trapped by the commitment I had made, trapped by the romantic delusions of the last lonely months, and embarrassed and angry at his unwillingness to trust these friends who had taken us in at a moment's notice.

On that bleak day in June, in all the desolate expanse of Europe there was only one redeeming feature, and that was Rosie. She must have been seven or eight at the time, still young enough to believe that the world revolved around her, and charming enough to ensure that it mostly did. And so she found it quite unsurprising that, on the day before her ballet test, a beautiful foreign dancer should conveniently arrive in her living-room. He should give her a lesson, she said, and help her with her preparation. She left him no choice. I watched as he began to instruct her, the white gold of her hair bobbing against his golden black, and I saw that her confidence warmed him, made him supple, and seemed to release in him a flow of irresistible grace. It was though I saw the life in him returning. It lasted no more than a few minutes, no longer than the span of her concentration. Then, when the dancing stopped, the chill crept into him again. And at night, when we went to sleep in the front bed-room, illuminated by the cold reflection of the cathedral floodlight, he would not let me come near him.

We decided to return to London, but the execution of even that simple operation proved unexpectedly complicated. Arriving late at the station, we leaped into the train at the last minute and found ourselves heading for Nottingham where they insisted that, if we wished to proceed to London, we must pay another full fare. An hour later, as we settled into the unheated carriage and the dismal prospect of Nottingham faded from view, with Juan defiantly playing his Walkman at full blast, the brightly anticipated reunion of our summer holiday was reduced to a moody snarl. It was as though, in the few months we had been apart, we had shrivelled, contracted into ourselves, so that we no longer connected.

Back in London, I called a former colleague who was working at the British Library, cataloguing eighteenth-century French pamphlets. It was the worst possible moment. Normally imperturbable Jim, the only man I knew who conducted interviews with vice-chancellors in bare feet, was morosely licking some emotional wounds of his own. The idea of playing host to Juan cannot have been very appealing, and Juan made no attempt to hide his misery. He was bewildered, tense and sickening now with the first signs of bronchitis, which is how I left him in Jim's flat in Brixton.

*

Berlin. Does the train still come in so slowly to the Zoo station, arcing on the elevated rail past the last stucco facades of Charlottenburg? Does it stop at all? Or does it now, at the end of its long haul from the Hook of Holland or from Paris, rush through to the Friedrichstrasse in the heart of old new Berlin as though no Iron Curtain had ever intervened?

Even to ask these questions is painful; they shatter the illusion that somehow the past can again be visited. I have perched on the low wall of the town square of Guantánamo; I have retraced out steps in the streets of New York; I have returned each year, when All Souls' Day comes round, to the grave. But the Zoo station?

Ten years ago it was firmly fixed in the permafrost of the Cold War. It was of one piece with a world in which Brezhnev still exercised his senile despotism over an evil empire and Ronald Reagan was re-writing the script of world politics in the spirit of Steven Spielberg. I do not recall thinking anything like this as I waited, once again, on the platform. If I had, I would have been better prepared for Juan's arrival.

No English summer could account for the beeswax pallor of his face as he bundled his bags, with exaggerated difficulty, down from the train. He looked as though he had caught a glimpse of hell. It dawned on me then, with a pang of guilt, that he had: at the border crossing, where the guard towers were hidden not quite discreetly enough at the edge

of the forest, and where the East German passport con-
trollers—always politely sinister—entered the train to
administer their temporary terror. Of course, nothing had
happened. Nothing except a rush of panic as he recalled the
water and the night of Guantánamo Bay, as he watched them
leaf through his second-class passport with the problematic
words 'Claimed Nationality: Cuban.' Had he really returned,
of his own free will, to the nightmare world of the
Communist International?

If he was ever going to relax in a holiday mood in
Berlin, it was clear that we would first have to neutralise the
Cold War. He was still wary, turned in on himself and
uncharacteristically quiet when we set off, at his request, to
confront the Wall. He disliked walking. 'These legs were
made for dancing,' he once protested when I was too mean
to hail a cab. But this day he walked purposefully, striding
through the Tiergarten and pausing only briefly to inspect
the toilet block that had achieved international exposure in
the gay film *Taxi zum Klo*. Then we were at the Wall and
on the viewing platform. To the left, on our side of the
Wall, was the Reichstag; straight ahead, on the other side,
the Brandenburg Gate with the famous Quadriga, reposi-
tioned so that the backsides of the bronze horses addressed
the West with a permanent fourfold fart.

For a long time he said nothing. He simply stared into the
East. Then a coachload of American tourists arrived. Where
were they from? 'Atlanta.' 'And you?' 'New York City,'
said Juan. One of the women repeated the news to a friend
who had missed the momentous information. New York.
New York. Like a magical incantation the words seemed
to reassure him, to establish firm ground under his feet, to
animate him. He was an American on summer vacation.

'Let's go, Johnny, let's go!'

We were not finished yet. Instead of turning back through the Tiergarten, he started out along the Wall to the south, pausing now and again to touch it, to read the graffiti, to control, to check, I thought, that the Wall would hold. By the time we were nearing Checkpoint Charlie he was beginning to romance about it, eagerly pressing me for more and more escape stories. How I had acquired such a stock of anecdotes I cannot imagine, but they surfaced in my memory now. In the early days people had simply escaped across the low barbed-wire barricades that were strung up along the border streets. Then, when the Wall went up with its four metres of concrete slabs rounded off at the top with concrete piping, they had tunnelled beneath it, or, more spectacularly, abseiled across it on ropes from the windows and roofs of adjoining houses. At particular transit points they had crashed through it in coaches and ambulances and delivery vans, until the guard was reinforced and the approaches made more deadly. More recently, two East German families and their children had breezed across the border in a hot-air balloon and landed, if you could believe the photos, trilling as blithely as the Trapp family singers.

We poked about the museum at Checkpoint Charlie, and watched the trickle of visitors disappearing through the checkpoint into the labyrinth of control posts on the other side. At an *Imbiss* near the Kochstrasse *U-Bahn* we bought a *Curry-wurst* and Coke and then retraced our steps—Juan insisted—back to the Brandenburg Gate. He was mellower now, and slipped his arm under mine as we walked—an unusual gesture for him in public. By the time we reached the viewing stand, the last coach parties of the day had been and gone. We stood together on the platform, and in the early evening light two rabbits appears in the no-man's land of the death strip. 'Bunnies!' he said, which, as far as we were concerned, finished off the Cold War.

I had rented a shabby ground-floor apartment in the Fasanenstrasse. This street name must have been the first German word that Juan learned, and he pronounced it with an explosive stress on the second syllable, so that it came out sounding like a trumpet blast, as though it were the proudest address in Berlin. In fact, the house was decidedly substandard, one of those turn-of-the-century speculative grey barracks built around a dank courtyard. In the spring I had been surprised by a thin burst of blossom from a couple of lilac bushes; otherwise there was nothing in the courtyard but metal rubbish bins and a permanent smudge of black dust around the coal cellar.

Our apartment had obviously been subdivided, possibly at the time of the postwar housing crisis. The bedroom and living-room were separated by a thin wall of plasterboard, and the kitchen was a niche carved in turn out of the living-room. This meant that the main room, still preserved in the original dimensions, was the bathroom, which boasted an enormous bath tub with magnificent claw feet and talons. This met with Juan's instant approbation; he made the room his own, and he stocked it with Oil of Ulan and balsam shampoo and aloe shaving lotion and threw out my Wilkinson Sword razor blades and replaced them with Gillettes. Into this steamy sanctuary he would disappear for what seemed like hours at a time. Now and again I would hear snatches of song and then, increasingly, the strange sound of German words and phrases being rehearsed: *Ach so!*, which he contrived to pronounce like a stage Chinaman, or *Fasanenstrasse*, with the trumpet effect. But mostly he practised the *ü*-sound, as in *Führer*, and *Türken raus*! which he had seen daubed on the Wall, and *Kurfürstendamm*. He found this sound both irresistibly comic and elusive. He seized on a line from the German version of *My Fair Lady*, and the bathroom echoed raucously as he sang it again and again: '*Es grünt so grün wenn Spaniens Blüten blühen.*'

Then, in a New York Spanish version of Henry Higgins' English: 'I think she's got it. My God, I think she's got it.' And then off again, as the bathroom swelled and crashed with much splashing for the grand finale: '*Es grünt so grün* . . .' Berlin was going to be a success.

Whatever the case might have been in England, that summer the German sun shone warm and even, much as it must have done, I thought, in 1914. By the end of July they were watering the street trees. The manicured patches of beach around the Wannsee were covered with perfectly tanned bodies, and so, more interestingly, were the meadows in the Tiergarten. In the city on the Ku'damm, as the afternoon wore on, elegant people appeared in the cafes, or walked their Dalmations, or gathered under the umbrellas at the tables on the Olivaer-Platz. It was perfect weather for *flâneurs*, perfect weather for Juan.

That the Ku'damm is vulgar is one of those rare propositions on which old-time Berliners, world-weary academics and idealistic youths who had moved to Berlin to escape the draft would all agree. By common consent it had become too plastic or, from a different point of view, too brassy. There was too much naked money and too much dressed-up sex to spend it on. There were too many tourists, drinking *Berliner Weisse* made pink with a shot of raspberry syrup, crowding into the dubiously Argentinian steak-houses, and endlessly consuming monuments, ruins, cakes, coffee and *pommes frites* with ketchup, with hardly a pig's knuckle or a plate of honest sauerkraut to be seen.

Wherever the real Berlin was to be found, this was real enough for Juan. In the course of his daily promenading, he proceeded to establish several vantage points from which he could view the street at leisure. One of these was the window table in a tea shop where the menu, if that is the word to apply to a list of teas, was as long as the Twining's catalogue. After you had ordered, the *Fräulein* brought your teapot to the table with a personalised alarm clock, timed to the exact infusing requirement of your preferred tea. If, as sometimes happened, two or three alarm-clocks went off simultaneously, the tea-room, which was otherwise as solemn as a dentist's waiting-room, suddenly resembled the workshop of a mad bomber. Precision tea-drinking, Juan decided, was one of the great German contributions to the serious art of living.

At the other end of the street he discovered a bench well placed to give him a view of an equally thought-provoking spectacle. It was opposite the square behind the Kaiser Wilhelm Memorial Church, a much-photographed land-mark that played host, no doubt reluctantly, to a permanent assemblage of punks. Be-ringed, be-razored and enchained with the same attention to detail as the precision tea shop, they seemed to have taken over the square as an outdoor living-room. With their shaved or hennaed heads, and their faces grey with the pre-putrescent glow that is produced by a prolonged diet of vegetables and dope, they com-plemented beautifully the grotesque Gothic ruins of the church. Sooner or later, if you waited long enough, a van-load of policemen would arrive, and after a token struggle and a volley of mutual insults, the square would be cleared.

The afternoon performance was complete, but to not to worry, said Juan, they would be back tomorrow. And they were.

La ronde: each scene in this self-absorbed world was entire in itself, yet endlessly repeated. Later, when we reminisced about Berlin, he remembered the fat woman with whom we were on nodding terms at Mario's ice-cream parlour where she came, as we did, for her nightly indulgence. 'Three flavours,' she always instructed the waitress, 'with mixed fruit and cream on top.' And there were the old ladies, with their mannikin hats pinned primly over their thinning silver buns, wearing their perpetual widowhood like members of a dedicated order. And in the evenings the little bar, intimate with pink curtains and a soft glow from the trimmed lampshades, where the boys sipped white wine and menthol cigarettes, and sighed tragically over the impossibility of finding a real man.

In the bar there were free copies of a magazine. It was called the *Berliner Anzeiger*, a very decorous title for what was really a monthly guide to gay Berlin. The August issue led off with an article on the Royal Porcelain Factory. There was an illustration of an eighteenth-century tea and coffee service, and under that a brief item calling for action against 'the new diseases'. In America, the article said, these new diseases turned up mostly in the leather scene, and now they were appearing in Berlin. Kaposi's sarcoma, and something else called GRID. It was nearly a year since I had read about the violet spots, but GRID?

'Do you know about this GRID?' I asked Juan.

'Yes,' he said, 'it's the gay cancer. People are talking about it in New York. It's really hitting places like the Mine Shaft. Only the crazies want to go there any more.'

Had he ever been there?

'No,' he said, 'you know I'm not into that scene.'

It was such a slight conversation. In fact I only recall it because he kept the August copy of that magazine as a souvenir.

He also kept some coloured catalogues from the KDW, the Berlin equivalent of Bloomingdale's. This was the domain of Martin, whom he had spotted one afternoon in the crowd on the Ku'damm. They had danced together in New York until Martin had moved for a while to the ballet in Stuttgart. After that he had pitched up, temporarily out of work, in Berlin, where he now presided with much zest and coppery-black good looks over the tropical fruit department at the KDW. As the summer trade in tropical fruits was lethargic, there was plenty of time for gossiping, and Juan took frequent advantage of this civilised way of conducting business. One day when he was happily immersed in conversation with Martin among heaps of jackfruits and pineapples and potted display palms, he was approached by a customer who presumably had equally little to do with her time.

'From which country are you coming?' she enquired in English. Professionally alert, Martin intervened in his best jungle voice, 'We are from Africa, *gnädige Frau!*'

No doubt she recalled the demonstrations by Somali wood-carvers and Bedouin leather-workers with which department stores periodically promoted their ethnic wares. Gesturing at the mounds of fruit, she asked, 'And are you part of the demonstration?'

'Oh no,' said Martin, with sad eyes and still deeper tone, 'We are for sale!'

That was our Berlin, our island in the sun.

Back at the Zoo station, with his two-day transit visa to Paris and a bottle of KDW perfume in his bag as a present for Hiram, Juan hugged me goodbye. We didn't kiss. Two men couldn't kiss in public. I knew he thought that. Not even on the Zoo station.

*

Shortly before Christmas I was back in New York, making a brief stopover on the long way home from Berlin to Melbourne. Juan had arranged to sub-let Danny's apartment during my stay. This was a mutually acceptable arrangement because Danny spent most of his time at Hiram's on the top floor of the same building, and there was no point in his paying out good rent simply to provide a home for the cockroaches. So we moved in, and out—while Juan set off a double-strength roach-exterminating chemical cocktail—and in again over the bodies of a thousand dead *cucarachas*.

We were back on 14th Street, not a stone's throw from the chapel of Our Lady of Guadaloupe with her Aztec halo. On the block nothing much had changed: the shoe shop, the drugstore where they sold conditioner for Afro hair, the Spanish bookstore with its sun-bleached posters of Gaudi's Barcelona church in the window, the haberdashers that smelled of linen and lavender when you pushed through the door. And near the corner, an Irish bar—the Shannon? the Shamrock?—with a sour smell that made Juan wrinkle up his nose as he passed, a remnant of an earlier era marooned now in a sea of Spanishness.

Off the street, though, and in the places where gay men congregated, there was a mood I had not known before. While Juan and I had been in Berlin, the homosexual cancer and the violet spots had acquired a new name. GRID had become AIDS. It still sounded strange and it was clumsy on our lips, and, especially here in New York City, it generated apprehension and confusion. When we discussed the situation with Danny in Hiram's apartment, it was his anger that impressed me most.

'They want to close the bath-houses,' he told me, 'and that will be just the beginning of a witch-hunt. If they get away with this, next they'll be burning faggots in the streets.'

'I think so too,' said Juan, who generally deferred to Danny in political matters, except where Israel was concerned.

It is tempting to think that the publicity about AIDS contributed to a small domestic drama that was about to break over us, but I am inclined to think that this was not the case, for the woman who provoked the unpleasantness appeared to maintain perfectly peaceable relations with the other gay tenants in the building. It was only to Juan, and by extension to me, that she directed her malevolent attention.

Presumably she had a name, since that is a requirement of the law. But no one appeared to know it, and she guarded it with the secrecy that other people reserve for their tax affairs or their criminal record, which frequently amount to the same thing. Not that she would have paid much in the way of tax. In the summer she read tarot cards in the Village, in a shop so narrow it was little more than a wall-to-wall wall. In the winter she appeared to hibernate and to retreat into the fastness of her apartment which, unfortunately, was directly below ours.

On a few occasions we had observed each other frostily in the elevator. Then late one night, she announced herself with a loud thumping on her ceiling. Juan was watching yet another re-run of *Dr Who* on the television and I was trying to sleep when the thumps came persistently under the mattress on the floor. Juan retaliated, hammering the floor with the heel of his Mexican boot. There was evidently a history to this relationship. For several nights the attacks, as we came to think of them, continued, always around the midnight hour with which, as Juan observed, she seemed to have a particular affinity. But the Mexican boot produced its effect and she subsided, as we hoped, in defeated silence.

On Christmas Eve she resorted to a new stratagem. We had been shopping at Balducci's, an extravagant gesture that pleased Juan. I had imagined we might come home with a turkey and an English plum pudding. But turkeys were for Thanksgiving and Juan didn't care for plums, so we arrived back at 14th Street with a new Christmas menu in place and ingredients to match: shrimps and prawns and clams for a *paella* and a strawberry shortcake in a box and a bottle of pink champagne. Then, along the length of the doorstep, as I fumbled for my key, we noticed a trail of white powder.

'Salt!' said Juan.

'But why would we have salt on our doorstep?'

'The bitch,' he exclaimed. 'She's into magic!'

'She's what?'

'Johnny, I'm sorry. You don't understand these things. We have to piss it away.'

It was true that I didn't understand, but I could see that he was in deadly earnest. There are times when loyalty requires that you do the strangest things. And so, clutching the strawberry shortcake in one hand and directing my penis with the other, I stood beside him pissing away the salt, until it washed down the hallway in a briny stream. But this was, after all, New York, so when the magic was thoroughly dissolved we mopped it up with paper towels and dispatched them down the rubbish chute.

Later in the evening she was back, snooping outside our door. Juan sensed her, and when he blazed into the corridor shrieking and bellowing and threatening to wring her neck, she fled to the elevator at the end of the hallway. Providentially—or was it rather due to the counter-magical power of our mingled urine?—the elevator door closed before he could make good his threat, and she was gone.

Against my better judgement, on Christmas Day in the morning we made a start on the strawberry shortcake. Then I slipped out to the corner shop to buy some bay leaves that we needed for the *paella*. In the ten minutes that I was away, two policemen arrived, and when Juan answered the door they twisted his arm and forced him against the wall and searched him, and told him that they were going to charge him with harassment. Wasn't it true that he had threatened to kill the nameless woman from downstairs?

We went up to the sixth floor for a council of war with Danny. Danny said that it was only her word against Juan's, but she was a middle-aged single woman, even if she was hysterical, and he was a young black Hispanic man, and a faggot, and it was obvious whose word they were going to believe. Hiram, looking slinky in a silk kaftan that might have doubled as a negligee, thought we all needed a *caramelo* that he had prepared in little porcelain bowls in honour of 'my' religious festival. In the end, Danny decided we would have to file a counter-charge of harassment against the woman.

At the police precinct, when we turned up around lunchtime, they seemed to be having a quiet day. The officer at the desk had his feet up and his jowls down and he was not interested. When we persisted, he turned preachy and gave us a burst about the spirit of Christmas that was the most self-serving sermon I had ever heard. But Danny wouldn't stand for that nonsense.

Even with his grey beard and his long plait, he looked tough. He talked tough too; not aggressively, just enough to show that he wasn't going to budge one inch. And perhaps the officer could see that he was Jewish and that Christmas didn't cut much ice with him. You are not supposed to notice things like that but people do, the same way we noticed that the cop was Irish. So finally he bestirred himself and produced a form to fill in.

The *paella* never got made, and when we came home to the apartment a new generation of chemically immune cockroaches was deeply into the cake. We bought a pizza and polished it off with the pink champagne.

Two weeks later the case came up at the community conciliation board. A nice black woman heard their stories. I'm sure Juan didn't tell her about the magic. Or about his lover who was here from Berlin. He was too shaken up to explain how hard he had worked to persuade Danny to let us have the apartment, and how he had looked forward to being the perfect host. And then that woman had needled and provoked him and fired him up and sent the police after him as if he were some mean street kid. That was what he hated most.

The conciliator listened to what they had to say. Then she pronounced the verdict that in future the woman was never to speak to Juan, nor he to her. Of course, the justice of this ruling could be disputed, because it was the woman, after all, who had started the affair. But Juan could live with it.

And besides, in a couple of days I would be leaving for Melbourne and Danny would be resuming his apartment. And Juan?

'Don't worry about me, Johnny. I'll be OK.'

CHAPTER FIVE

But miles and miles away
Suffers another man.
He was young, open-hearted,
Strong in mind and body
When all these things began.

—Anthony Hecht, 'Three Prompters from the Wings'

For the next three years we lived our lives on a kind of instalment plan. We had times together, and times apart. In Juan's case, you could say that the pattern of his life resembled an airline schedule, or the indicator board at an airport with the destinations flipping over as the planes arrived and departed: JFK-LAX-SYD (was this stopover really necessary?)-MEL. Four times he came, and then a fifth. And because the efficient operation of international travel presumes a tidy predictability that was quite alien to the forces that governed Juan's life, there was always drama.

The problems began, once again, with the visa. In the laminated offices of the Australian Consulate-General in New York, they received his application for a two-month visitor's permit graciously enough. But unlike the Dutch, who had issued him with a travel permit in the previous year as though he were a normal person, or even the Germans, who had required only four weeks to investigate his suitability to visit Berlin, the Australian authorities would not be hurried in the meticulous execution of their duties. After several weeks they were still unable to inform him when his case might be decided, and when he pleaded that the departure date for his non-refundable 'Apex' flight to Melbourne was fast approaching, they reminded him that he ought not to have presumed on receiving a visa in the first place. He phoned me from the lobby in the Rockefeller Building in despair. It seemed that he would not be coming.

It is a formidable thing to tangle with the Department of Immigration. Naively, I expected a well-mannered call to their local office would resolve the problem. They referred me to Canberra, and when I spoke to the people there, they vaguely referred me to New York, as though it were so remote as to have passed beyond the bounds of all accountability. Undaunted, I contacted New York, where they informed me that personal representations at the Embassy in Washington might be necessary: and in Washington they referred me to Canberra. The due investigative processes appropriate to the granting of a visa must run their course, they said, though what that course might be, or why the running was so slow, or to what end the investigative processes were directed, they were unable to say, because that was the responsibility of their officers in New York.

Their system was perfect, their defences impenetrable; except that they failed to anticipate the intervention of my friend Paul, the most bureaucratically insightful person ever to be unemployed by the Public Service. He read and marked their regulations, including the smallest print and the most subordinate paragraphs, as fast as they could produce them, and he devoured the contents and relished the plots of pamphlets on civil rights with the enthusiasm that other people reserve for detective novels. He was a model citizen, a tireless advocate of rights—civil rights, gay rights, workers' rights, tenants' rights, the rights of pedestrians and the rights of the unborn. This, he agreed, was a difficult case. 'Nevertheless,' he said, 'you must phone the Ombudsman, and insist on your rights.'

Did I have a right to be visited? I had no idea: but the Ombudsperson agreed that I certainly had a right to be angry. She was sure, she said, that there was no prejudice at work in the case, but she would take up the issue as a matter of urgency. Within hours she produced results, and there was a reverse-charge call from Juan in the Rockefeller lobby on Fifth Avenue to confirm it. They had called him in to collect his visa, and in eight hours he would be on his way.

As we discovered when we went through this farce for a second time six months later, his mysterious difficulties had to do with the fact that his 'claimed nationality' was Cuban. He was therefore, according to the logic of the Department, possibly a Communist, and as a Communist he was a possible threat to the national security. It is not easy to prove that one is not a Communist, and it is even more difficult if one is never asked. And unlike the Americans, who were very good at asking this question of their intending visitors, the Australians, being a polite people, preferred to avoid such a confrontational approach and to conduct their enquiries more discreetly. No evidence of Juan's subversive inclinations came to light, but in its researches the Department did acquire an important piece of information—presumably from the FBI—that led them to doubt his integrity. Did he stand by the declaration he had made routinely to the effect that he had no criminal record? Of course he did. Then why, they wanted to know, had he concealed his encounter with the police on a certain evening in February 1972? They had lighted upon the saga of the cockroaches in the Greenwich Village restaurant!

This time we knew the routine. I poured out the story to the astonished Ombudsperson and explained how Juan, though still technically Cuban, had long since embraced the attractions of bourgeois individualism to which in any event he had been predisposed ever since his grandmother had pressed him fresh guava juice in Guantánamo, and how, if you thought about it, this was perfectly consistent with his determination to eat a cockroach-free dinner in the restaurant with the priest. The Ombudsperson agreed and, drawing on the remarkable plenitude of her powers, once more she intervened, and once again the officers in the Rockefeller Building were required to reach reluctantly for their visa stamp.

'It's time, Juancho,' I said to him when he arrived for the summer and we were lying on the beach at Wilson's Promontory undermining national security, 'it's time that you got yourself a proper passport.' 'Yes,' he said, 'I'll have to become an American.'

Between our hard-won holiday reunions, we kept in touch by phone. And there were letters. He didn't normally write letters. I never saw him write one, not in all the time we spent together. He called people up, and if they were out of town and not at home, they might as well have ceased to exist. But to me he wrote. It was never a regular flow, the kind of exchange you could describe as a correspondence. The letters came helter-skelter, sometimes two or three a week and sometimes none for a whole month, but they were always rich with his moods and his voice—like this one that he wrote after his first visit.

New York City
9.17.83

My dear Johnny,

How are you? I mess you very much. My impretion with Australia are really marvellous. Beside been sick for so long, I am still bother by this terrible 'itch'. It have not going away yet and is driving me crazy.

Things are just exactly as I left them, not much change. They all envy me. For New Year Hiram have a dinner for some friends from his church plus Betty and her husband. After they all got drunk Betty said that she can't stand it that I have been all over and plus I'm going to have a degree from college and who do I think I am. By that time I was making believe I was sleeping, so they continue and I stay on my own thinking about you and Australia. Papy, how I feel I could just quit everything and disapere. I did not mess New York one bit when I was there with you.

In later years we wondered sometimes why it was that Australia seemed to make him sick. On that first trip it was Bell's palsy. We had been to see a movie in Carlton and then dropped into Genevieve's for coffee. As we came out he stopped on the corner of Dorrit St and complained that the left side of his face was frozen. By the next morning it had subsided into a kind of mongoloid droop and the doctor, who valued an open relationship with his patients, thought it appropriate to warn him that in twenty-five per cent of cases the treatment for his condition would not succeed. This time it did, though agonisingly slowly, and then it was followed by an outbreak of shingles that raised little pustules of concentrated itchiness across the small of his back. The medical dictionary we consulted concluded its brief entry on *herpes zoster* with the comment: 'Has been known to drive people to suicide.' So it was small wonder that in his next letter he confessed to having been depressed.

9.28.83

My dear Johnny,

Your letter arrived just on time to cure me of my acute depression.

You are very correct my dear. To me the best time we have ever spend have been in Melbourne. Every-time I hear something or see something from Australia I feel some kind of knot on my chest and I feel home sick.

By now you have seen the newspaper clipping from the much talk about victory in 132 years. I'm very happy for Australia. But for a moment it was 3-1 America and after that the rest is history. The media have gone crazy because they could not believe after 3-1 they could lose and they lost. The beauty of.

The completed sentence, I suspect, would have read: 'The beauty of it is that these crazy Cubans, who always put me down and tell me that Australia is unsophisticated but are really intensely jealous, are taking the Bond victory as a personal affront. On the other hand, thanks to Mr Bond and his punching kangaroo, my stocks have never been higher!'

There was good news, too, on the job front. He had been interviewed for a part-time job as a booking clerk with the People's Express Airline.

There is only one catch: I must have a 'suit' . . . So I am depress for a suit because I want that job, so please I'm ask you to send me some money to buy me a suit right of way. I am very excited about the job. It was $5 per hour with benefit of free travel anytime anywhere but it does not go to Australia.

Papy, I feel O.K. now because I won't be any more walking the street. I may rent a furnish room in a cheap place so I can save some money for my trip to Australia in Dec-Juany. Right now I don't have a cent, and I need that suit before class starts in 3 weeks. The rule says: 'Business ataire' (suit, shirt and tie).

Fortunately he was able to beg or borrow a brown reefer jacket with gold buttons from a friend, which apparently satisfied the sartorial expectations of People's Express. They took him into their training programme almost immediately.

Every time that I walk into the centre, I feel nervous and a beat ashame for not having some good clothes. The training is for two weeks and with one week pay if the test is pass or no pay if the test is not pass and of course NO JOB. I'm scare of not passing the test.

He passed the test, gratefully pocketed the one week's pay for two week's work, and settled into a routine that was arranged for the days when he was free from college classes.

At the end of the year, before his second trip to Melbourne, they assured him they would hold his position until his return, but when he returned their circumstances had changed and his services were not required. And so, when their circumstances changed still further later in 1984, he reported the matter with some feeling:

10.11.84

Ah, a big scandal just happen with 'People Express'. Well it was in the news for almost 'slave driver.' 527 people quit their jobs. All students. Because with students and no union those people were exploited and if you complain you were fire on the 'spot'. I was shock when I saw the news. They too were guilty for no hiring disable or fat people, so is good that the city got in their 'case'. How about that?

Indeed. But although there was some satisfaction in seeing the airline exposed, this did nothing to solve the problems of their erstwhile employee. He was surviving in temporary accommodation in a welfare hostel.

I still very unhappy with no job. Living out of suitcases really bother me. The hotel is full of 'roaches' everywhere. Smell terrible. I have my stuff in a locker in Penn Station because I know somebody was in my room. Nothing was lost but still is a welfare hotel with all kind of people. $65 a week for that 'shit'. I who had an apartment for more than 11 years with all my things to nothing is very very depressing.

Well, I mess you very much and everybody too. Every small thing like songs and movies etc. that I saw there really send me back to Melbourne. That is crazy because I don't feel like that any more for Cuba.

Take care. Kisses and hugs.

And remember that I love you very much.

Juan G. Céspedes

In fact he was no longer sure where he belonged. He had recently become an American citizen, and though the primary purpose of this step had been to secure an American passport in order to circumvent the complexities of travelling to Australia, paradoxically it also meant that he was now free, at least in theory, to visit Cuba, a country to which he was by no means as indifferent as he sometimes pretended. That was evident in his next letter.

I send the $42 for my 1er U.S. Passport that will make me feel legalized not only but secure. Now I know I will have no more trouble with 'visa' or 'nasty Germans' like in London. That I can go to Cuba too. That really is the icing on the cake. My terror is over and so my nightmare of been deported to a hustla country like Cuba.

Meanwhile, he took seriously his new status as an American citizen. After the presidential election in November 1984 he offered this analysis of the results:

Well, all is over and we still have the same President, like I told you and Murray one day in the house. I feel sorry for Mondale for the way he lost. And how he lost. Reagan won every state in the Union. People don't forget how Carter and Mondale did not do much for the hostage crisis. He was in China and Germany and the Philippines to mention a few country and what happen? 444 Days of Degradation for the U.S.

You might think how American I am. Well no, I'm still the same. The citizenship have not change my view about this country, but I have rather be with Reagan than Mondale. Only for the record of both man.

This last comment was intended, I imagine, less for me than for Murray, a witty left-wing law student whom he had come to know in Melbourne and who teased him about his hawkish views. I was less concerned by the return of Reagan than by other snippets of more personal views.

Enough of politics. You know what is happening here. Well last week I was sick with a cold just like the one in Ingland. My chest was falling off and it hurt. Winter is here and very strong already. Is heavy coat, ah, tell Murray that he give you the pattern to make a coat, or get the name of the pattern at Michael's Courner Store they have it because I want to make a coat for winter.

He survived the winter and in February 1985 he arrived in Melbourne for his fourth visit, this time with a six-month tourist visa that they happily stamped into his brand-new US passport. I hoped that on this visit he would make up his mind to stay—not that it would be easy to secure permanent residence, but there were encouraging straws in the wind. A Human Rights Commission that had been investigating discriminatory practices in the Immigration Department had recommended, as I learned from the gay rights grapevine, that discrimination against homosexual couples should be removed. This Minister was supposed to be sympathetic, but after the election in December 1984 there was a Cabinet reshuffle in which West was replaced in the Immigration portfolio by Hurford, and there was much anxious holding of breath in the gay lobby. A Catholic family man, they muttered darkly, as though the Pope himself were about to insert an infallible finger into the local political pie. But the signs from Canberra continued to be encouraging and slowly, with no fanfare, a new and more liberal policy seemed to be taking shape. The real danger was the possibility of adverse publicity, which we feared might be orchestrated by the more troglodytic elements on the Opposition benches against a background of mounting AIDS hysteria. But the news circulated only in whispers, and the flood of opposition that we anticipated never broke.

Despite the opportunity opened up by this change in policy, Juan was not yet ready to commit himself to stay. He wanted to come: he was thirty now, and at thirty part of him wanted to become a settled person, with a home, where he could look out the window and watch the passing scene from inside, where he could meet someone and invite them in for a meal and tell them casually, 'Of course Johnny won't mind. He always cooks enough for three.'

But he also knew there would be a cost, and it was a cost he would never cease to pay. He had learned that in America, even though New York—at least from one point of view—was almost an extension of Cuba. Cubans had always gone to New York. You could move in and out of the Cuban crowd twenty times a day. They knew where you were from and who you were. And even if they gave themselves airs and graces and told stupendous lies about how rich and important their families had been before the Revolution, that was also part of being Cuban. Or at least it was part of being a Cuban refugee.

But in Melbourne? Here they couldn't even pronounce his name. He was like an exotic bird, the only one of his kind. And though occasionally I thought he was over-sensitive, I couldn't deny that people did look at him in the tram and in the street. They did stare. They would have touched him if they had dared, reached out and run their fingers through his hair to see if those wet curls were real. At the market the Italian girls on the fruit stall saw him coming; they waited for him every Friday afternoon. 'Michael, Michael!' they squealed, because they thought he was a Michael Jackson look-alike. Of course that was before Michael Jackson whitened his face and became really strange, and the Italian girls meant it as a compliment, but we re-routed our shopping expeditions and went down another aisle to avoid them.

In the end it was not the distance from Cuba and not the thought of Michael Jackson that decided him. He was not quite finished with New York. He would go back one last time. With one more semester he would be able to complete his college degree. That was important. To be sure, it would not be the prestigious uptown piece of paper that Marymount issued to its graduates. They had finally terminated his scholarship in 1983 when his grades and his attitude had been deemed unacceptable. But a poor person's degree from the Borough of Manhattan Community College was still a degree, and although they had no dance programme, he responded enthusiastically to their courses in travel and tourism, and discovered in himself an unexpected ability in biology and maths. Twice he had made the Dean's List with three As.

And so, after a six-month break, he was back in New

York City at the end of the northern summer, and the 'my dear Johnny' letters resumed.

> I really don't know how to beginning. People were in shock to see me because if you deasapeared is because you catched AIDS. So Hiram was very indifferent to me, plus I did have to pay him some $. My friend Jerry that I was keeping while sick didn't let me a cent for all my work. That too is nasty. Still I did not espect anything, but some of the people who never were around when he was dying of AIDS got his condominium and car and other assect. Well, some are like that.

Jerry? Did I know Jerry? I had become used to the ways in which Juan compartmentalised his life, and I had learned to be content with the information he volunteered if and when he considered it to be appropriate. It would not apparently have been appropriate for me to know then—as he told me later—that Jerry had had sex with him even when he knew, as Juan did not, that he had been diagnosed with AIDS. Not that it would have made much difference to our sexual behaviour. We had discussed the question of infection several times. My attitude was fatalistic; we had been together now, on and off, for more than four years, and if there was any infecting to be done, it must surely have happened long ago. But in the last few months Juan had insisted on some minimal precautions. Was Jerry the reason for this—poor, rich, inconsiderate, dead Jerry?

Apart from the affair of Jerry, there were other frustrations now that he was back at college. The complications of his degree had long since left me hopelessly baffled, but I understood at least his disappointment when they told him that he would not be able to complete his degree, as he had anticipated, in one more semester. There were certain of his subjects at Marymount for which they could not grant him full credit and, in particular, he would still be lacking English I.

The lack of English I paled into insignificance compared with his lack of a home, his lack of money and his lack of luck. He had rented a furnished room from the low-income housing authority in the City, but for this they charged $79 a week, 'so that I won't last long in there,' he wrote:

So far not even work I have and no money either. Your $200 went to pay 140 for part of the tuition; TAP award me only $512 of $612, plus $39.50 of activities fee. So there you have it. And I'm not counting three books I have to buy but I have to wait until I get some kind of work.

I'm free from classes M.W.F. to work. Have gone down the Village and made some store give me some applications for job, any job. I called People's Express Airline and I still waiting to hear from them. The rats! I'm waiting to hear from a health food store run by some Hare Krishna set. The interview was very well, but nothing either. Tomorrow I will pass by again and see if the position have been fill.

I'm not very well. I have lost all the weight I came in with and more: in total 14 pounds. The heat is murder, the streets are full of people practically naked, man and woman no exception. I am running like a chicken without a head. Nothing seem to click.

And to top it all, last week was the biggest lottery ever in the US or the world for that matter. '44 millions.'

91

I still can't believe the numbers were: 4-12-28-32-41-44, suppl 39. My # 5-12-27-33-42-45. I cry for at least an hour. I can't believe still of how close I was. I still have the ticket to prove it.

He was plainly homesick now for Melbourne. Letters came with unprecedented frequency, always finishing with the command 'Write! Write! Inform me!'

Tell me more of how everybody is doing. Even Father Foster. The Brady, the chucks, the peacocks, and of course Albert and please don't cut off his balls. Have you seen Brent? Or Murray? I really mess everything and everybody, so make sure and tell them. Have they ask for me? And you, Papi, are you working in your books? How are they doing?

It should perhaps be explained that I—we—lived in a block of four flats, a solid thirties construction of clinker brick, and spacious as such buildings go. Our immediate neighbour on the ground floor was Father Foster—the Rev. John Augustus Cory Foster to be precise, which is necessary to distinguish him from me. In a lifetime of frugal and dedicated service to the Church, Father Foster—now well advanced in his eighties—had allowed himself, as far as anybody knew, only two passions: he was devoted, with more or less equal ardour, to the English cricket team and the work of the Foreign Missions. If anything upset him more than losing the Ashes, it was the sight of coloured men, as he called them, arriving as refugees or immigrants to take up residence in this country. It was, he said to me with high indignation, as though they thought they had a right to be here. 'We took them the Gospel,' he said, 'and now they come and perch on our doorstep.' The mysterious comings and goings of a coloured man in the next apartment must therefore have been a matter of some annoyance to Father Foster. Had this fellow not received the Gospel in his own country? And yet, with the passage of time this unnatural order of things grew to be familiar, and the familiar came to seem natural; so natural, indeed, that now and then there would be a tap on the back door, and Father Foster would appear with a tray of apple tarts or mince pies fresh from his oven. 'The young man might like one,' he would say; though in view of the unusual odours emanating from the old priest's kitchen, the young man generally declined.

Beside our flats was the house of Father Jim, the parish priest, and beyond that was a bluestone church, a modestly pleasing Victorian pile in a style that might best be described as family Gothic. Together with the tennis court and kindergarten and the adjoining gardens, this compound provided an ample home for a constantly growing menagerie. The first animal we had acquired was Albert, a marmalade kitten who had emerged from the chemistry cupboard in the convent school where the priest's wife was employed. This unusual beginning in life left Albert with a permanent neurosis and a standoffish disposition for which the cure, according to Juan's diagnosis, was fatherhood. Consequently, on his next visit, we acquired a second cat which Juan bore home in triumph from a neighbourhood alley and christened 'Victoria'.

Then there was the peacock. With this creature Juan developed a special affinity, even to imitating its distinctive gait: the sharp forward thrust of the head and neck and the cumbersome gathering-in of the body, as though when it walked it were rehearsing the memory of its own serpentine evolution. During its first few weeks in the compound we had kept it in the chookhouse, and when the time came for its release, citing the authority of his dimly remembered training at the Veterinary Institute, Juan took charge. To prevent it from wandering he tied a long string around one leg and attached the string to a plum tree, but it promptly tangled itself around the tree and burst into such a honking and shrieking that Albert shot up a pear tree, and Father Foster appeared in his doorway speechlessly flailing his arms and looking as though he would like to despatch both Juan and the bird to the nearest mission. A Cuban peacock might stand for this kind of treatment, but clearly for this one a different approach would be required.

This was the community about which he was so anxious to be kept informed. Well, I replied, for the moment the peacock was doing nicely, though it had recently paraded in Queensberry Street and brought the traffic to a halt. Father Foster was fine. Murray had got a good result for his thesis about the dingo which did or did not eat the baby Azaria and would be writing soon. Phips, the Old English Game bantam had taken ill and died, and Prizzi, Juan's rooster, which we had had to despatch to a friend in the country, had unfortunately been eaten by a fox. Finally, Victoria had produced five kittens under the kitchen sink. As the enclosed photographs showed, all were doing well, except that one had an infected eye.

This assorted zoological news was well received, and there was a reply by return mail.

9.22.85

I was very pleased with your letter. It was so beautiful
to see my 'babys'. She looks so motherly taken care of

her babys. It bad that one is sick. Take much care and make sure is not contagious at all. How is Albert looking at fatherhood?

Sorry about the chuck but I told you they must be check by a vet.

Farmyard talk was a welcome diversion from his own troubles.

Me, well, that is another history. I had a minor triunf in school: but no luck with work. Too many promises and that's all. I have failed so many applications and nobody have come true. That is now getting depressing because I'm broke. Practically stuck in one place. Now any fare unpaid and they stop you is 3 months community services. Is that I'm not into that!

So there. Just make sure you prey for me, please God! I'm really down and I don't know how long I can take this shit.

Between writing and posting this letter his fortunes and his spirits lifted. As always happened when he was really distressed, or really excited, he put through a reverse-charge call to me. In these urgent moments time zones meant nothing, so I was frequently asleep when the unpredictable calls came through and was sometimes a little slow on the uptake. Or, in fairness to myself, I might say that it took a while to adjust to the tumbling sequences of his narrative. And so, after the phone call, he added a PS to the letter.

'John,' it began, which sounds as though I must have been particularly obtuse that night. Or did this solemnity

mark the joy that he felt in recovering in himself something
that he had mourned as lost?

> John, what I was saying is that I will be dancing in a
> new company directed by Alvin Ailey who's main com-
> pany was in Australia in Augost last. Is the second black
> co. of New York City.
>
> Well, the program is made of dance from his reper-
> torio and is called 'Dance Search' because its main goal
> is to seek out new talents in Junior High, College, etc.
> So we'll be dancing in auditorio around N.Y.C. We
> will hold master classes to see who has talent so they
> can be properly place in school around the country. So
> I think is great. They ask me where do my training is
> from and I told from 'Cuba' and they were very please.
> I will have the chance to choreograph or teach; what-
> ever I want to do. Only problem—no money involved.
> Is only 'experience gain,' but in my case I'm delited
> because I have not dance in 2½ years.
>
> I'm sore in both legs, but O.K.

From Melbourne I also had encouraging news to report.
In August I had been to a meeting to discuss the problems
that gay couples were still encountering with the Immigration
Department. Out of this gathering there emerged an organi-
sation which called itself the 'Gay Immigration Task Force'.

We were the oddest collection of bodies, united only by
our same-sex preference and a common yearning to enjoy
the monogamous comforts which the rest of the population
found so constricting. In this circle, as I recounted to Juan,
there were people in every conceivable conjugal state. There
were two lesbians from Berlin: one had married a local man

in order to qualify for permanent residence and the other, who had a botanical name I am inclined to think was Poppy, with hair to match, was well advanced with a similar marriage plan, which she hoped now might not be necessary. Next there was an Australian man of indeterminate years who had married an Englishwoman as a favour, and was now seeking a divorce so that he could apply for permanent residence for his diminutive Indonesian (male) lover. An older businessman from the outer suburbs was desperately in love with a Filipino boy to whom the Department had refused even a tourist visa. A self-effacing Jewish man who had dealt with the Department over Jewish immigration problems was there to give us his advice but not his name, because a gay identity was not considered an advantage in communal organisations. Finally, there was a West-coast American with that confidential tone of voice that translates so successfully from the seminary to counselling, and his local lover. They had met in Japan, and the American was here on a six-month tourist visa. 'I'm going to keep in touch with them,' I wrote to Juan, 'because they seem to have their act together, and their case is not so dissimilar to ours.'

By October I was able to report that the GITF was making progress. The West-coast seminarian had been to talk with the Minister in Canberra and brought back details of the new arrangements. The Minister was willing to admit gay partners of Australian citizens who had been in a continuous relationship for four years. More than that, in the case of more recent relationships, a gay partner might come on a visitor's visa, which could be extended every six months until the four-year point was reached. 'Under these guidelines,' I wrote to Juan, 'you could apply for permanent residence the moment you come back, and unless there is some terrible political upheaval in the meantime, it should be more or less automatic.'

I was assuming now that his decision was made. He replied:

10.15.85

My dear Johnny,

Your letter sound so good that I will not believe until is official because sooner or later it will be known all over Australia. But I think that is great that finally some high ranking official understand our cause.

Today I had good news from school. It is true that I will receive $1,005 from the Pell Grant. I must say that I'm very delighted. I doing very good in school. In the 1er of three tests done already I have in Maths 94, French 88 and in Chemistry 82.

I'm feeling much better now. My stomach is back to normal, but now is winter and, well almost winter, and already is been at freezing point some knights and I only have the long coat. I don't have a jacket. I left them there. I should have with me the grey leather one.

The stomach worried me. For weeks—or was it months now?—he had been complaining about a sore stomach. I tried to persuade myself that he was being alarmist. On the other hand, those terrible itches had not been imaginary; the little lesions on his back and buttocks that left the brownish spots were not imagined; and nor were the bronchitis and the racking cough and the loss of weight. I must have discussed these things with Murray, who alluded to them in his next letter, which received the following response:

My dear friend,

Your letter was so cheerful that I give it to other people to read so they can laugh too.

I'm not sick, and I do eat a lot. N.Y.C. may be a dump to much people who have never been there. But tell me where in the world you can go at 4AM in the morning and buy a pastrami sandwich? Definite not Rusia!

Well, I'm happy that you are keeping in touch with Johnny. I think he needs company from time to time. We are in touch almost every week. I call him at almost any hour.

You don't know how much I want to be there and see my 'children' playing in the garden and see them grow. I think that I made a mistake but that was some-thing that I had to do, so I know what I really want. Now my mind is clear. No more pain in my chest. And my memory is just, well, just that. A memory. I'm free.

Do you know John is coming to N.Y.C.? He will be here for 2 reasons and I'm one of them of course.

My dancing is coming real fine. It been so long that I should be more rusty but I'm not. I'm sore from head to toe and my leg is not as high as before but it feel like I have never stop dancing. Plus Alvin Ailey's Co. is one of the biggest modern dance co. in America, so maybe that makes my adrenaline flow with more zest. I'm very happy. Delaighted.

The performances are in December. John will be here by then. He have seen my choreography but I don't think he have seen me dance. That is mainly why I'm doing it, and for me too.

I never did see him dance. Between October and December there was a hitch in the arrangements with Alvin Ailey. Did the funding dry up? His disappointment was so keen that he didn't want to talk about it or even, on this occasion, to bemoan his luck.

CHAPTER SIX

I am like a flag surrounded by distances.
I sense the winds that are coming, and must live them.

—R.M. Rilke, 'Presentiment'

I flew into New York with the snow. Five years earlier, on my first visit, I had detested the worn-out February snow, packed hard and piss-stained where a thousand dogs had walked their owners on the streets. It had seemed like a two-toned city, yellow and grey like the ribbons that had still been fastened to the street trees to celebrate the release of the Middle East hostages and the end of '444 days of degradation'.

This December snow was different. It was falling softly as we drove from La Guardia airport across town to the studio apartment on Riverside Drive that Juan had sub-let in my name. The key wouldn't turn in the lock and we had to fetch the doorman to let us in. He was a young Puerto Rican, sleekly pleased with himself in his braided uniform.

'I hope you'll be happy here, sir,' he said to me, as though Juan did not exist. 'You'll like the view.'

It was late afternoon and the sky in the west was already dark. To the left of our window the George Washington Bridge thrust out over the Hudson. Straight ahead, the cliffs of New Jersey rose sheer from the river; there was nothing but winter trees and snow and the powerful grey river, and no sign of humanity except for the chain of light where the traffic flowed noiselessly across the bridge. The vast silence of the scene impressed me. Standing behind me and looking out over my shoulder, Juan slipped his arms around my waist.

'Did I do good?' he asked.

'Yes,' I said, 'you did fantastic!'

He had a Christmas present for me. Shouldn't we wait till Christmas? No, no, he wanted me to have it now. It was a 'Movado' watch, the only watch, he told me, that was in the Museum of Modern Art, the perfect design. It was a beautiful present, and a great compliment, really, to the Pell Grant people who had made it possible.

That night I had diarrhoea. Squatting on the lavatory bowl I had time to admire the watch on my wrist and to notice how it nestled in the hair that grew more thickly on my forearm than almost anywhere else on my body. And to wonder. This business with my bowels was no more than a traveller's accident, the result of a germ picked up from a ham sandwich or the tropical fruit, perhaps, that I had eaten at Honolulu airport. But Juan also had diarrhoea. Not the spectacular 24-hour variety that kept me up all night, he explained, but loose, half-formed and so persistent that his arse was sore.

AIDS? We skirted round the word, assuring ourselves that he had no fever, no night sweats, no violet spots, in fact nothing more serious than a slight acid feeling in the stomach and loose bowels. And of course he had always been prone to that problem and had always had a low tolerance for milk. Cheerfully seizing on that fact, I suggested—though I was hardly convinced—that a more sensible and regular diet might settle the problem. He played along with this strategy and so we agreed, at least while we were in New York, to augment our diet with *plátanos*, but boiled rather than fried, and spiced with lashings of garlic and lemon juice. Green *plátanos* would gum up the bowels of a duck.

The green *plátano* cure was sufficiently effective to allow life to continue normally. Back at the German-Jewish archive I was immersed in a new accession of documents that promised to reveal the remaining secrets of Hans and Klaus. Juan was doing exams, for which he prepared in the evenings, sitting upright on the floor with his legs spread at an angle of ninety degrees and his notes conveniently assembled between them. The day the results were to be announced he insisted that I come with him down to the college on Chambers Street. We were early, and whiled away the time buying Rastafarian Christmas cards from a stall, watching an inter-collegiate netball game, and marvelling at the information provided in the college handbook. The campus, situated on 4.28 acres, was a $128 million megastructure that was equivalent to the Empire State Building lying on its side (minus the tower). We had an interview with a course adviser, who said that Juan's course was now complete with the exception of English I and that he could complete that for credit at any *reputable* university in Australia. Was the English Department at Melbourne University reputable? They would have to check it out, said the adviser.

His results in French and chemistry were posted on a board and were most satisfactory. The maths result would be announced in class by the professor, who turned out to be a diminutive Chinese woman with spectacles so large that they framed her cheeks as well as her eyes. The students, apart from an almost white Argentinian book-keeper who sat to one side of the room in a kind of self-imposed male reserve, were largely Haitian women in varying degrees of middle age; and there was Juan, the only 'A' student in the class. The book-keeper, I thought, looked slightly peeved at Juan's success, but the women squealed and applauded and embraced him and wondered how he could be so brilliant. The Chinese professor made a little speech in which she thanked the class and said they had all worked hard and that they all congratulated Juan on a great result and wished him a very happy life in Australia. She was sure, she said in the nicest way, they would need mathematicians down there. The farewell rituals had begun.

In the weekends we went out to Queen's to visit Ernie, the businessman who sold sporting goods and equipment for gyms and who was the most enduring of Juan's succession of patrons. In a fix, he could always be relied on for a meal and a bed. I suspect that is how Juan had survived the last semester, though he had had to make do with sleeping on the living-room sofa because the spare bedroom was occupied by a Puerto Rican boy from the Bronx whom Ernie had taken in when he was in trouble with the courts. Juan didn't care for him much; he considered him a sly little queen, which he probably was, though even sly little queens deserve a go.

Everything about Ernie was solid: his house, his furniture with its heavily timbered and padded look, his considerable frame, his conversation, his cooking. He specialised in shepherd's pie, which Juan found boring, though I secretly approved of these calorie-rich, bowel-stopping dishes with their three-inch crust of mashed potato.

For all his paternal affection for young Latins, Ernie inhabited mainstream America. He lectured Juan from time to time about getting a full-time job, perhaps as a salesman in the men's department at Macy's. That particular suggestion was received with speechless disdain which turned into a torrent of protest the moment Ernie was out of earshot. Didn't Ernie understand, after all these years, how important it had been to finish his college degree? Did Ernie really think that he was good for nothing but selling briefs in a cheap department store? Well, perhaps not. At any rate, when he wrote a reference for the Department of Immigration in Canberra, he put things in a different light. It had been his pleasure, he wrote, to have known Mr Céspedes for approximately twelve years. 'I first came to know Mr Céspedes when he acted as a Trade Show adviser to this Company, assisting in the design and set-up of New York Trade Show displays. During this time he proved himself to be talented, dependable and a positive contributor to our success.' He was certain that Mr Céspedes' character and intellect would make themselves quickly known wherever he might be.

Meanwhile, Ernie wanted to give him a parting present: a bike. One Saturday afternoon we drove out to Long Island and pulled into the carpark of a suburban sports store. It was just after Christmas and they were doing a lively trade in exercise machines. We watched the antics of a group of women in designer tracksuits, who were looking for a machine that would trim their post-festive flab with the greatest speed and the least expenditure of energy. They called each other 'you guys', and giggled and hooted and chattered at the top of their voices and hardly seemed to notice the price tags. Suddenly we were in middle America. Was it this that made Juan uneasy? Or was it simply the huge array of bikes of every conceivable style and make, so that choosing *one* was as difficult as buying a salami in a Berlin sausage shop? German or Hungarian? With pepper or without? With the pepper inside or outside? How should he know? So he stood in the middle of the showroom looking dazed, and assented gratefully when Ernie took charge and settled on a grey and pink machine with a German-sounding name and more gears than there are hills in San Francisco.

We had leased our room with the view on Riverside Drive for three months. I intended to leave in mid-February, and by the time I was back in Melbourne my next salary cheque would be enough to cover Juan's fare. We called at the Qantas office and waited till the black woman was free and booked him a seat for the end of the month. Then he began to bargain with me. Couldn't he leave a bit earlier? Did I really need another four weeks at the archive? Was it absolutely impossible to find the money for the fare before the end of February? This was not the gamesmanship he employed when we negotiated a movie to see or a friend to visit. He was urgent and quiet. And although he would not say as much, I knew that he wanted to see a doctor, and his doctor was in Melbourne. So we did what I had sworn was absolutely impossible and brought forward my departure date by a month. After I had been to the bank manager, he would follow two weeks later.

On our last day together in New York we went down to the Village, feeling nostalgic and planning to have lunch at the Pink Tea Cup in Bleecker Street. It had moved, gone up-market and trebled its prices to pay for the new pink linen tablecloths. We sauntered along 14th Street and lit a candle in the church as a gesture of thanks to the Lady with the halo of Mexican daggers. Crossing the road we called in at Hiram's so that I could say goodbye and Juan could use the loo.

Last of all, I said goodbye to Ernie. 'Take care of the kid,' he said, as though he were entrusting his son to me. I liked Ernie. But about Juan and me, I thought, Ernie didn't quite understand.

CHAPTER SEVEN

'The slight despair
At what we are,
The marginal grief
Is source of life.'

—W.H. Auden, 'The Exiles'

We were not like lovers in a novel, amazed with joy in the moment of our reunion. We had travelled too often, and too far, for that. No, it would be truer to say we were content, happy with the prospect of ordinary pleasures and a life together. And if we had known how brief this time would be, how fragile were the foundations of our contentment, we would not have arranged things any differently.

He arrived on a visitor's visa, as the GITF recommended. We seemed to fit so neatly into the Minister's guidelines that we didn't anticipate any problems with his application for permanent residence. The only cause for apprehension was the health tests the Department routinely administered. Would they introduce an AIDS test, either as a general policy or, still worse, targeted at high-risk applicants? There was pressure for them to move in this direction, though so far they had been deterred by concern about civil liberties or the desire to maintain the confidence of what they now described increasingly as 'the gay community'. Yet if they did introduce the test, what if he turned out to be HIV-positive? Would they declare him a public health risk? Would they consider the care for him an unwarranted impost on the national health budget? Would they send him back to New York? And then? The sooner he submitted his application, the better.

By now the GITF people had considerable expertise in the matter of applications. They had advised on half a dozen cases and the Minister had complimented them on the exemplary documentation provided. Clearly it would be wise to follow their guidelines.

In submitting an application they said, the Australian half of the committed relationship needed to show that if the permit were not granted he would suffer severe emotional hardship. But how do you talk to a bureaucracy about such things?

It seemed easier, safer, more in line with the GITF's sense of etiquette, to leave my threatened emotional stability to the representation of friends: of Susan, who had opened her house to us in Lincoln and guided us round the cold cathedral; of Jim, whom Juan always associated with the great bearded Assyrian kings in the British Museum; of Rickard, to whom I had first written about my encounter with Juan; of our neighbour, Father Jim. They composed the most supportive testimonies, saying that we had been through thick and thin, that it was costing us a fearful amount of money to maintain our trans-Pacific relationship and that I would suffer severely if the Minister didn't give us what we wanted. The combined effect of these statements was to make me sound a trifle unhinged; but Juan thought that they were perfectly correct.

There was a lot that was left unsaid. Take the question of money, for instance. There were people who wondered about that. They asked me, 'Who paid for all those fares?' And in the end, when it was all over, I was even asked, 'Who paid for the grave?' Well, of course I did. Nobody said it was a scandal, not directly. But you could tell from the way they narrowed their eyes and said 'Oh!' that they were busy making moral calculations, about Juan, and about me.

We weren't embarrassed about money, except that there was never enough. In fact, money was a subject that I had always found profoundly tedious. With the comfortable security of a tenured job and the luxury of having no dependants, I had never given it much thought. In mildly profligate reaction against the thrift of a middle-class upbringing, I spent what I had, or I gave it away, and the savings that had still mysteriously accumulated had gone to pay for that un-salaried year in Berlin. This indifference to money—or this irresponsibility—was a trait in me of which Juan entirely disapproved, and when it came to paying for those airfares and subsidising various expenses in New York, I began to see his point. It was rarely so easy as simply writing out a cheque. To raise the cash for one airfare I had to sell an antique book-case. It was an *art-nouveau* piece, but I had come to dislike its swirling lines and was happy to see it go. I had no compunction either in selling a mahogany pedestal desk. It looked magnificent but was never used because I preferred to work on the floor, so the removal of the desk was pure gain.

It was different with the icon, the Russian icon of Our Lady of Sorrows that hung over the mantelpiece. I *was* attached to that. But if it was necessary, as once it seemed to be, I would have sold that too.

'No,' said Juan, 'you must never sell the icon.'

'Never?'

'No,' he said, 'not even for me.'

No one could predict how long it might be before the application was processed. In the meantime Juan was not entitled to work, so that he was thrown back completely on his own resources. Sometimes, when the weather was still warm, he would cycle to St Kilda where he liked to see the palm trees, or to South Melbourne beach where he was more diverted by the bodies. In more pensive moods he walked in Royal Park, or he would turn up unexpectedly at the university for an early lunch which inevitably became a late lunch. Or he would step out, as he put it, to visit Murray, who lived in a glorified lean-to which a Maltese family had tacked on to the back of their West Melbourne terrace. The approach to Murray's place was through a cobbled lane, and the longer Murray lived here, the more attenuated the lane became. Removing one bluestone pitcher after another, he transformed it into a garden, and the success of this original landscape became, in Juan's mind, the yardstick for our own. He was beginning to enjoy his patch of earth. Next summer, he said, we would grow tomatoes.

During the day mostly he occupied himself with sewing. His aunt had been a famous seamstress in Cuba, he once told me, as if to imply that this was a family skill he had inherited along with his curls and his fine long fingers. He had sewn theatre costumes in New York, and taken courses at the CAE in men's tailoring and fashion design, and there was no doubt about his proficiency. On one of his previous visits we had bought a Janome sewing machine which soon began to produce a stream of shirts and trousers all carefully copied from the latest Italian designs in Collins Street shops. While he sewed, he sang, lustily and out of tune, though this hardly mattered because his voice could scarcely be heard above the blast of the cassette recorder that sat on the corner of his cutting table. As often as not these unrestrained sewing binges brought Father Foster banging on the back door in protest, but that hardly mattered either because his protests were generally drowned in Juan's creative cacophony.

The sewing began to take on the dimensions of a cottage industry. There were curtains for the flat, cushion covers for parish ladies, and a couple of skirts in red tartan for a forlorn little girl called Gypsy whose mother was preoccupied with writing poems about Auschwitz. Juan's public reputation as a tailor rested on the grandest undertaking of all—the project of the purple banners. The need for these arose because a new assistant bishop had been appointed, and to welcome him to our local church a splendid liturgical reception was prepared. In the midst of the choral rehearsing and floral decorating that the occasion required, Juan applied himself to making banners, six swathes of discounted purple cloth from Michael's Corner Store, each twenty feet in length and appliqued with the bishop's insignia in gold lamé, which were to hang down the Gothic pillars of the church. They looked spectacular, and the bishop was sufficiently delighted to join us in the evening at an impromptu dinner party in a Turkish restaurant.

Recalling his earlier episcopal encounter in New York, Juan approached his second bishop as something of a connoisseur. He particularly admired the bishop's ring, a large stone set in a broad band of gold that was made from the melted-down wedding rings of his divorced admirers. The practical consecration of their sorrows in this way made the ring an object of general interest, and it was passed around the table from hand to hand until Murray, who was present on this occasion more in the category of the poor than of the faithful, accidentally dropped it in a dish of eggplant dip. There had been a time when Juan would have been appalled at such a gaffe. Now, he was more forgiving. After all, he observed to me later, Murray was not in the habit of dining with bishops!

After the banners came the quilt. Naturally it was not *the* quilt. We didn't know about that then. We hadn't heard that there were men in America sewing their own memorials; that there were lovers and friends patching together their grief and their anger, and conjuring memories out of the most incredible collection of things—letters and sequins and flags, and names and dates, bits of clothing and even ashes, so that you could no longer distinguish between art and death; and that when their separate sorrows were joined and the quilt grew large, they would spread it out in an enormous field, and soon there would be no field that could contain it.

We had no reason to be thinking about memorials, and so it was mere coincidence that Juan began to make a quilt. Like the coincidence of being born under the star of that abortive revolution; or the coincidence of arriving in New York in time for Stonewall. It came about simply. He was passing the Meat Market Craft Centre one morning, and stopped to inspect an exhibition of quilting. Being the only visitor, he fell into conversation with the exhibitor. A country woman from Bacchus Marsh with straw-blonde hair and pink cheeks, she was charmed, I like to think, by his courtesy, or perhaps she simply responded as a dedicated quilter to a potential convert. In any event she sold him her book on the subject and signed it with all good wishes. In the book she explained that she had been quilting since she was knee-high to a grasshopper. Patching and quilting her way through life, she had always used traditional English and American designs until, in the sleepless nights when she was expecting her first baby, she had been inspired with a vision of new motifs reflecting her Australian environment. Instead of the Churndash and Clay's Choice and Log Cabin and the Variable Star, she had thought to herself, why not the Desert Pea Whirl, the Waratah Wreath or the Banksia Bouquet? *Patches of Australia* was the result, the indispensable guide to Australian quilting.

Having gutted the book for its essential techniques, Juan was now contemplating a quilt of his own. Happily impervious to the design potential of his Australian environment, he was equally indifferent to the subtle gradations of muted colour that refined taste prescribed. His quilt would be a blaze of clashing, flaring colour. 'Hot, hot, hot!' he told me, as he picked his way through the remnants of cloth on the stalls at the Victoria Market. Ideally, his quilt would be so bright you would need sunglasses to look at it. What, after all, was the point of having colours if you didn't use them? And without use, might they not fade away and leave you stranded in a nightmare world of olive drab and salt-bush grey?

Progress on the quilt was slow. This was understandable because, although he didn't have a lot to do, he had a lot to think about. About Hiram and Danny, and about Julio and his friend David, to whom he rarely wrote though, in a curious way, that simply increased the need for thinking. He thought about Cuba, especially when the ABC presented a naive report extolling the achievements of the Revolution and the way it guaranteed first-class medical treatment even to the poorest of the poor. If that was the case, why was he receiving requests from his mother to send pills for her heart because, she wrote, they were not available in Cuba?

And when he thought about hearts, he remembered Clara de la Rosa, whose heart he had broken and who had died so soon after his flight from Cuba. For more than sixteen years, more than half his life, he had lived with his remorse, until, quite without warning, he decided on a course of action to assuage his guilt. Would Father Jim say a mass for his late grandmother? He would: and so we gathered in the church and lit the candles and rang the bell, and the priest made a sacrifice of bread and wine, and prayed that the Lord would open to Clara de la Rosa the gates of paradise where there was no death but only lasting joy.

Quite without warning—that was how it seemed. And yet, later I discovered it had not been an impulsive act. In fact he had written to Cuba and received from his mother the exact date of his grandmother's death. Then he had waited for the day when the anniversary returned. How precise, how proper, and how silent he could be!

Having done what he could for his grandmother, he had more time to think about his own future. About himself there was a mystery. He was not sick: but neither was he well. The old soreness in his stomach persisted and his bowels were still loose. At each visit to the gay doctor he lay on the couch and slipped down his underpants, and the elegant medical fingers in latex gloves glided over his body, probing, pausing over the swollen lymph glands in his groin, and finding nothing. The doctor always chatted. He cooed gently like a dove. Was the diarrhoea worse or better?

Well, Juan would say, as though he was trying to encourage the doctor, he thought it was a little better. And of course any precision in respect to this question was impossible. How do you describe the infinite gradations that are possible in the viscosity of excrement? So, although he was generally a little bit better, he remained a little bit sick.

One day the doctor said, 'And have you been out dancing, Juan?'

'Not much,' he replied.

'Why is that?'

'It's that Johnny isn't into discos much.'

'Johnny ought to take you dancing more often.'

It's surprising the things you learn at the doctor's. Though I made no comment, I bridled at this gratuitous advice. It reminded me, though less acceptably, of Ernie's parting words, when he said, 'Take care of the kid!' They both saw in him the boy. They seemed to think that all he wanted was to be a son, to be looked after. Of course there were times when he did want that. But taking care cuts both ways, and at home they would have seen that a more complex order of things prevailed. Since Juan had arrived there was an order in our house that had not been there before. The rooms smelt more sweetly. The spices in the kitchen cupboard were all lined up and stoppered and labelled, and really contained what the labels said. It was becoming the kind of place where you wanted to be sociable. And when you went out, you had the feeling that you had lost that single look. Maybe we should have gone out more often. And maybe the doctor was speaking out of the kindest consideration, but he didn't know how happy it made us to be at home.

On our next visit to the surgery—Juan always insisted that I accompany him—there was another prescription for more pills. As they were likely to be expensive, the doctor suggested that we might like to take the prescription to the dispensary at Fairfield, where we could obtain them free of charge. For this kindness Juan was grateful, so it seemed churlish to mention my own reservations. It seemed odd that we should go to Fairfield; there were other public hospitals much closer to home, and in a penny-pinching mood I calculated that the cost of the taxi fares would cancel out any saving on the prescription. Nevertheless, we couldn't play with his health; if it was necessary to go to Fairfield, we would go. The next morning we ordered a cab and drove out through Northcote, past the beat where a young man had been poofter-bashed to death a few weeks earlier, and pulled up at the gatehouse of the Hospital for Infectious Diseases.

My own memories of this Edwardian institution were decidedly romantic. It was some years since I had been there during a bout of hepatitis so mild that I had vaguely enjoyed the chance to be an invalid and to lie on my bed reading, without the guilty sense of wasting time. As I had discovered then, Fairfield was surrounded by extensive grounds and gardens that rambled down to the river. From a horticultural point of view they were badly neglected, but I had been delighted to find a suckering patch of *romneya*, a kind of perennial poppy with huge heads of white petals and gold stamens.

Superimposed on this recollection of Fairfield as the home of the great white poppy was another image. The out-patients' waiting room was a light spacious place, surrounded with long windows that opened out on one side to a covered garden of semi-tropical foliage. In the ceiling there were fans with long blades that turned slowly to move the summer heat. It was a pleasantly lethargic room, the sort of place where you half expected a Singapore waiter to glide up and offer you a gin sling.

The morning we arrived, as I noted with approval, it seemed even more exotic than I remembered. On one side of the room the benches were occupied entirely by Vietnamese: thin men, and women in St Vincent de Paul clothes, and red-faced squawking babies. TB patients, I presumed. On the other side, where the tropical foliage grew, was a bench of rough, tough younger men in tight jeans and tattoos, who produced a collective impression of smudged black ink. Hepatitis cases? Bikes and boat people; the place smelt of raw poverty, of welfare, which was explanation enough for Juan's instant recoil. Refusing to sit in the waiting-room, he propped himself against the door jamb in a truculent pose and silently directed his fear and resentment at me for having brought him here.

The receptionist feigned indifference to our unspoken altercation. After half an hour of waiting, after I had explained for a third time that we had not come to see a doctor but needed only a signature on a prescription form for the dispensary, she finally relented, allowed us to jump the queue, and ordered us into a small cubicle with a desk and two chairs. On one of these a doctor immediately took up her position of command and indicated to Juan to take the other chair.

'And who are you?' she said to me. When I had explained she ordered me to sit down, so I sat down in the only possible position, on the floor.

Looking directly at Juan, she began bluntly. 'I want to talk to you about AIDS.' She paused, perhaps to gauge his response, but Juan deflected her gaze to me. Feeling ludicrously disadvantaged from my position on the floor I replied as firmly as I could. 'I don't think we're ready to talk about AIDS. I mean, we just came to collect a free supply of pills from the dispensary. All we really want is a signature.'

It was abundantly clear from the way she sat back in her chair that she had no intention of releasing us. But why? What did she know about us? Why should she make these assumptions about us? Had the doctor with the probing fingers been in touch with her and turned over to her the delicate question that he had never broached with us? As these suspicions chased through my mind, she was well launched into an explanation of the virus and the high-risk category of gay men and the high-risk activities in which gay men indulged. As though we had recently dropped in from the moon, I thought. But she sailed on, explicit as you like, until she reached the point of her lecture: you should take the test.

Of course we had discussed taking the test. We had weighed the pros and cons, and decided not to. We knew that the chances of being positive were high, very high. After all there was Jerry, though we were disinclined to dwell on Jerry in this deathly speculation. Before Jerry there had been other men, in the Continental Baths, and at St Mark's, unremembered mostly, but any of them a potential source of infection. In New York City they were going down like flies. But wasn't it better to live with the uncertainty, to err, if need be, on the side of hope, than to live with the certain knowledge that you were going to die covered in violet spots? Like Jerry, and Rock Hudson, and all the others?

There was a more immediate, more compelling reason not to have the test. For Juan it had been important not to know when he filled in his application for the Department of Immigration so that he could say, as he did, and with a fair measure of truth, that he was in good health. There was no need to tell the Minister that he had loose bowels and a sore stomach any more than if he had had an ingrown toenail. So we had not taken the test.

The doctor insisted. She talked hard, working on Juan, and again he diverted her question to me. 'Well,' I said, 'there is virtually no treatment and no cure. What is the point of having the test?' And she—who was no doubt keen to establish the epidemiology of AIDS, and to monitor and control its spread, and to promote behavioural change and pursue a dozen other worthy socio-medical objectives—she replied, 'It will help you to plan your lives.'

Plan our lives? We could hardly believe it. What knowledge did she have that we did not? Was she pronouncing a sentence of death already? How long did she think we—or was it Juan alone?—might have to live? And how could we plan our lives while the bureaucrats in Canberra were not working on his application for permanent residence? We would have liked nothing better than to be able to plan our lives, but this was ridiculous, and I said so. 'I think so too,' said Juan, though I was unsure if he was really agreeing or simply supporting me in what had become a restrained confrontation with the doctor. By now she had exhausted her arsenal of arguments and failed to budge us from our position, and so she shrugged and signed the form for the pills and sent us off to the dispensary, where an artistic professor from the university was creating a scene because they had run out of free syringes. Near the gatehouse on the way out there was a border of evening primroses which had seeded themselves prolifically. We scooped up a handful and took them home in a plastic bag together with the pills.

The doctor had merely asked, 'Why don't you take the

test?' Yet her intervention was so unexpected, and she spoke with such force, that she had broken through the fragile defences of Juan's uncertainty and transformed his anxiety into a terrible conviction. What other explanation could there be for his malaise? There was no way the virus would have overlooked or spared him, not with his luck. 'Plan,' the doctor had said, but what should he plan when she had wiped out his future? Before the trip to Fairfield, however anxious he was, and however depressed he became because of the limbo in which he was having to spend this year, there was always the prospect of next year, and the one after that. And now? He felt dizzy, unbalanced, because suddenly there was no future to weigh against the present. He was like a man who has lost his shadow, weightless, insubstantial, and when I tried to reassure him he said, 'Don't touch me, Johnny. Don't touch me.' He was terribly afraid.

The virus makes you obsessive. It settles in your head. It distorts your vision. In the first flood of knowing—or believing—it can make you regard your own body with horror. The blood that is in you is lethal. It could drive you crazy if you dwelt on that knowledge, if you said to yourself, 'I am the embodiment of death.' Although those were not the words he used, it was clear that his thoughts were running in that direction. One morning he cut himself shaving. He wiped the blood off on a towel. 'Get the bleach!' he shouted to me in the next room. But there was no bleach, so he wrapped the towel in a newspaper and threw it out in the garbage.

We never returned to Fairfield. As far as planning our lives was concerned, we concentrated on getting ourselves to Sydney for a few days. The trip to Sydney is normally no more arduous than taking a tram to the city, but the night before we left Juan contrived to stand on a sewing needle and drive it into his heel. In the middle of the night we hobbled to the casualty department at the Royal Melbourne to have it extracted. When we arrived in Sydney he was still hobbling and it was still raining, as it had been on our previous visit. Then, we had laughed at the inconvenience, and imagined that Sydney would one day go the way of Venice, or slide off its foundations in a gigantic avalanche of mud and simply float away to sea under the Harbour Bridge. And the queens in Oxford Street discos would still be dancing. This time the rain was no joke. It was threatening, and for most of that week Juan holed himself up in the safety of the hotel TV room, warding off bronchitis or pneumonia or some other opportunistic infection that the virus was waiting to unleash.

Slowly the panic subsided. And the virus—if there was a virus—was so quiet that we dared to reassure each other with the possibility that we'd been wrong. It isn't easy to give up hoping. But I noticed that he was moving with less energy now, though he managed to mask his condition by playing on the image of the lethargic Latin. In June we went with Rickard on an expedition to Hanging Rock, for which Juan prepared with thermal underwear and a fleece-lined jacket. It was not exactly climbing gear, so when Rickard skipped ahead up the rock path, there was some excuse for Juan to trail behind, and to linger at the summit and wonder about the children who disappeared.

The signs were multiplying. A few days after the climb up Hanging Rock he came back from a trip to the local chemist dejectedly wheeling the pink and grey bike and leaned it against the wall near the front door. That was its last outing; he could no longer ride it up the Queensberry Hill.

And there was no denying the fact that it was now taking us twenty minutes to walk to the doctor, when previously we had covered the distance in a brisk twelve or comfortable fifteen.

The doctor prescribed more Lomotil for the diarrhoea, and more Mylanta for the stomach. He cooed with sympathy when Juan related the events that had taken place at Fairfield and suggested now an alternative. Perhaps Juan would like to consult a specialist in the gastro-enterology clinic at the Royal Melbourne. This, Juan agreed, would be sensible, because the Royal Melbourne was no more than a few minutes' walk from our flat, and there was a convenience store on the corner where you could buy a soda on the way home.

He weighed in at the clinic, rather light at fifty-five kilograms, and we sat—in the couple of hours I had free between classes—on the bench outside the consulting rooms and discussed the problem of his 'ulcer' with an Italian woman who recommended chick peas as an infallible cure. And then we were ushered into the presence of Dr Wall, who was neither smooth nor silky, but pleasantly avuncular and just old and silvery enough to give the impression of being infinitely wise. He explained that it would be necessary to do some tests, and of course it would be sensible to include an AIDS test because, as he was sure Juan understood, it was better to look at all the possibilities so we could get a proper handle on this problem. After the shock treatment at Fairfield, this advice seemed perfectly reasonable. The result, as he knew and we knew, was perfectly predictable. Juan was HIV-positive.

He received the news with a curious detachment. Coming out of the hospital, the first choice he faced was whether he wanted a can of Fanta or a can of Sprite, since Murray had long since shamed him out of drinking Coke. The next problem was whether I had time to cook dinner and still arrive at a public lecture on time to propose a vote of thanks. He phoned a taxi for me, and when I reached the venue I called the priest's wife, Ann, and told her his result. Would she mind calling in during the evening and spending some time with Juan until I got back?

The lecture washed over me. My mind was full of AIDS. Did the lecturer have an argument? Was she running a line that I should comment on? I had no idea. In proposing the vote of thanks, I wanted to confront the audience and demand to know how they could sit there so complacently when my friend, my lover, Juan, was dying of AIDS. Instead, I mumbled some forgettable words of appreciation, and when they moved on to a sociable cup of tea and buns, I phoned home. Ann answered.

'How is he?'

'He's fine,' she said. 'We're watching *Dynasty*.'

CHAPTER EIGHT

'And what of His sure mercies that He swore in the ancient days—where is His tempering for our bare back and sides—where is provided the escape on that open plain?'

—David Jones, from 'The Book of Balaam's Ass'

It could not be said that his condition was secret. Rather, it was simply private, in the way that so much about him was private. He preferred to listen than to talk, to watch than to be watched, except for those increasingly rare social occasions when he propelled himself on to centre stage with a burst of self-parodying theatricality. It is true that he was beginning to acquire the aura of an invalid, which is what happens when people repeatedly ask 'How *are* you?' with a meaningful stress on the present tense. But as his replies were vague and inconclusive, the world at large—insofar as it was interested in him—had no choice but to accept his fiction of the ulcer and to speculate. He confided in Murray and I confided in Ann and Rickard, and it helped to hear them echo back the assurances that we had from Dr Wall.

He did not have AIDS. Dr Wall was quite clear about that. He had the virus, and he had some specific complaints for which he took specific remedies: Fasigyn and Maxolan and other pills with equally meaningless names, names so devoid of fantasy that I was inclined to feel sorry for the disenchanted world of the pharmaceutical industry which invented them. Beyond prescribing these pills, Dr Walls offered no prognostications. He required no threatening plan for living, and his tactics and his temperament reinforced Juan's own inclination, after the initial shock, to let the morrow take thought for the things of itself. So there was no reason to abandon the dinner party we had planned for his thirty-third birthday and no, said Dr Wall, there was absolutely no prohibition against drinking French champagne.

With this medical imprimatur, which Juan interpreted more as a command, the small dinner party I had imagined, with four or five guests, expanded and began to assume the dimensions of a community feast. The guest list grew to two dozen, who could only be accommodated by clearing out Juan's sewing-room, borrowing some trestle tables and setting them up in the form of a capital E. We begged and borrowed chairs: Bauhaus tubular steel, Victorian rosewood, Viennese bentwood and canvas garden chairs smelling of winter mould, all of which created the impression of a furniture sale room, though this effect was adequately subdued by the starched damask tablecloths. In Juan's view these cloths, which came from the trousseau of an elderly German-Jewish friend, had class. He claimed the task of laying them out for himself, smoothing them down with the reverence that he reserved for objects of special quality: the Movado watch, the Russian icon of Our Lady of Sorrows, his own fur coat.

'Two meats,' he said, when we discussed the menu. 'You cannot have a feast without two meats.' I was sufficiently well trained to know that this meant automatically chicken and crackling pork. Then he added a third, a crown roast of lamb filled with apricot stuffing and cracked wheat. He detested the strong flavour of lamb. (Indeed the worst thing about Australian men, he once told me, was that they smelled like sheep, and I had wondered with a jealous twinge how many such men he had been on sniffing terms with.) The crown roast was there for its looks. The rest was pure Cuba: dishes of beans, plates of saffron rice, deep-fried balls of sweet potato that were supposed to come out of the oil with a crispy coat and a creamy centre. And *tamales*, minced corn that was heavily spiced and wrapped and tied and boiled in the corn husks like little green Christmas bon-bons.

The guests, when they arrived, were as oddly assorted as the chairs. Father Jim was there, and Ann, and Judith, the director of a local gallery. There were three or four gay couples, all on their best mixed-company behaviour except for Patrick, who had once sung in a church choir where he had acquired a repertoire of scandalous ecclesiastical jokes. Inviting Patrick had been a risk and Juan kept a strict eye on him because, as he explained to him in a serious talk in the kitchen, the guest of honour was a bishop, and he would not like the bishop to be offended.

This was Juan's third bishop, but unlike the others this was a real Church of England prelate with a seat in the House of Lords and a wife who was entitled to use the Lady Peeresses' room in the same establishment. Here, Juan learned with some hilarity, the peeresses retired as occasion required to perch on polished mahogany lavatory seats and to twinkle aristocratically into bowls of finely patterned porcelain. That was a piece of information he would store up for Hiram—if he should ever see him again.

In fact, the bishop and his wife were a modest couple. They were visiting for the wedding of their daughter Alison, and as she happened to live in the upstairs apartment, for a few weeks they became our neighbours. On the evening of the dinner the bishop was in an expansive mood, and after a sufficient drop of champagne he responded to Juan's entreaties to tell us, again, about his visits to Sandringham, and what the Queen had said to Prince Philip, and what Prince Philip said to the chambermaid. As the bishop launched with mock reticence into his recitation, Juan sat back in his chair at the centre of the capital E, relaxed and beaming at the unlikely moment of this command performance. It was as good as *Dynasty*, and hardly less consequential.

Reflecting on the birthday dinner I realised that if Juan were going to be ill, it would have to be a sociable illness. No dim lights, drawn blinds, closed curtains; no signs hanging for months on the front door like the one I had heard about in Fitzroy: 'Thank you for your visit but I do not wish to be disturbed.' On the contrary, he was hungry for company.

In the weeks following the dinner there was more than enough company and a positive whirl of activity as Alison prepared for her wedding. Alison was an action woman. She was forever skiing, bush-walking, riding, zipping around the outback in a two-seater plane or trekking through Indonesian jungles, which is where she had met Chris. But now that her jungle romance was to be formalised at the altar, she was plunged into an agony of indecision about such normally unproblematic things as dresses and shoes and bouquets. Although Juan had never been to a wedding in his life, he was more than willing to be drawn into the consultations that flowed up and down the back stairs, happily flipping through bridal catalogues over a cup of tea with the bishop's wife, and pronouncing as authoritatively as anyone else on the relative merits of taffetas and silks and brocades. Under the strain of these considerations the bishop's wife developed a nervous diarrhoea, and on this subject too Juan was in a position to give advice.

Juan would miss Alison and her homely, unaffected friendship. A couple of days after the wedding she and Chris flew out to Chris's home in New Zealand, and Juan returned to his interminable waiting. Sometimes it seemed that his whole life now was filled with waiting: waiting in the queue at the hospital (and no matter what time he made the appointment, no matter how early or how late, they would ensure that he spent most of the afternoon waiting); waiting on the virus that was in him, wondering how it would next announce itself and waiting, despite himself, for the first tell-tale violet spots; waiting on the Immigration Department, anxious for some finitude, some certainty or decision that would shape the shapeless passage of the days.

Each month we received a newsletter from the GITF. The list of approved applications was lengthening: Erling and Joe; Heike and Heather; Alan and Graeme; Victor and Terence. Why the delay in our case? Perhaps it had something to do with the fact that, according to the newsletter, 'couples where there is a wide age difference and/or cultural backgrounds may expect to undergo an interview'. Was nine years a wide age difference? Did Cuba make us eligible for an interview on the grounds of possible cultural incompatability, or did New York cancel out our cultural divergence? Or could this delay be accounted for by a continued hunt for evidence of Juan's subversive Communist connexions?

We wondered how we would handle an interview. I didn't like the sound of that word 'undergo'. The newsletter reported that Leon and Bhoy had been grilled for two and a half hours, separately and together. When, where and how had they met? Did they sleep together? What was their previous sexual experience (hetero and homo)? Was their relationship exclusive? Were they exclusively homosexual? Would they ever get married? It was good to be forewarned about the Department's questions though, as Juan pointed out, it wasn't terribly helpful if they didn't tell you what the correct answers were. We guessed, though, from the drift of the questions, that exclusive, pure gay monogamy was what they were likely to reward.

*

If that was what they were looking for, I wonder what they would have made of a letter that was sitting in the drawer of Juan's sewing desk. I came across it after he died. It was from Ronnie. Many years ago Ronnie had arrived from Israel to make a name on Broadway, and ended by teaching classes in college maths. Somewhere along the way, he met Juan.

New York
June 2, 1984

Dear Michel,

Hope you had a great trip to Australia and arrived safely. I want to wish you a good summer and hopefully you'll come back in good shape, anyway better than you left.

It's sad that our relationship had to come to an end on such a sour note, but I guess that's the way you chose to do it.

It was evident to me for the last two months that you either planned it to upset me, because I didn't give you enough money, or that you are so disturbed that I hope you'll seek some kind of psychiatric help. Your absolute refusal to discuss the reasons for your behaviour are puzzling to me. It's unfortunate that you can't, or don't want to verbalize your feelings. Every time I tried to talk to you, you didn't even want to listen. The TV was always more important.

I really don't think I deserved that kind of treatment and I am just angry at myself that I didn't put an end to it when you started your crazy moods. It is really hard to take.

I tried to help you a bit with my limited resources. But you never thought it's enough. Even our sex life became very monotonous and one-sided. To get a decent kiss out of you was like pulling a tooth, increasing my feeling that you really only wanted to use me. Your friend in Australia is obviously more important to you than I, which is O.K., but you should at least have said so and not act so nastily.

I am writing all that because you never wanted to listen or talk seriously to me. Anyway it's over now, and I hope for your own sake that you will make an effort to change.

I leave for Calif. in four days.

All the best, yours,

Ronnie

'It's an old story,' I would say to the interviewer if he had confronted me with Ronnie. 'Look at the date. Two years ago.' Yes, but what did this letter say about the claim that Juan and I had been through thick and thin together? What did it say about our claim on each other?

Well, I might have said, in a way I knew about Ronnie. There were letters from time to time, and when I asked who Ronnie was, Juan was vague. A friend. So I assumed there was probably some kind of sexual liaison involved. I would have preferred it otherwise. I might have been jealous, even angry, if I had known the details. But it was all very far away, in New York, and I didn't need to know. As for the sex, gay men have sex with other men all the time. No particular emotions are involved. You might consider that a scandal, or you might think of it as a kind of liberation, but the fact is, that is the way the gay world often works.

Of course this affair with Ronnie was more than a fleeting encounter, and it went on long enough for each of them to hurt the other. I regret that pain, and I'm sorry for Ronnie's bitterness. He clearly didn't realise that he was the latest in Juan's succession of patrons, a successor to the priest and the engineer. There was affection in these relationships, but from Juan's point of view they were never exclusive, or binding, or passionate. Ronnie didn't see that. He hoped for more, even when Juan tried to explain. (Why else would he have mentioned me?) They were caught in a tangled web, unable to manage their unequal desires.

If the Immigration authorities had known these things, I suppose they might have said to me, 'And what makes you think that you are any different from those other men? From Ronnie, and Ernie and the engineer? Why do you imagine he is committed to you?'

To that question I could only have said, 'Believe me. I know. Trust us.' What other guarantee could anyone give? 'Let's see how things turn out.'

*

It was six months now since Juan had made his application, and he was nagging me to phone them, just to see how the case was getting on. Thinking of the medical examination that would come at the end of the bureaucratic process, I shrank from hastening the day. In his condition he would never pass the check-up. He was obviously underweight, and though he cheated the hospital weighing machine by wearing a heavy overcoat and a pair of boots, the evidence of his decline was undeniable. Fifty-five kilos, fifty-four, fifty-two. For a couple of weeks his weight would stabilise, and then the process resumed.

At the end of August, when his stomach was not responding to treatment, Dr Wall decided on a gastroscopy. The results, like the results of the colonoscopy six months earlier, were inconclusive. On a sheet of hospital note-paper, Dr Wall stamped a diagram of a stomach that looked like a billabong in a particularly winding river of intestine, and annotated it with the words: '*No* ulcer. *No* cancer.' Beside a small patch he had marked on the lower edge of the billabong he wrote: 'Mild gastritis. The Ulsanic is good for this, so complete the course.' It sounded such a minor complaint, so manageable that it would have been churlish not to respond to his sensible cheerfulness.

But then Dr Wall had not been present in the day ward after the gastroscopy was completed. He had not seen the cleaners move in while Juan lay still drowsy on the bed; he had not seen how they moved quickly and nervously in their white masks and gloves, swabbing and sweeping and even vacuuming the holland blinds and pronouncing him with their rituals of hygiene to be a leper, a plague-bearer, a polluted being.

'Do they normally do this?' I asked the nurse.

'They have their job to do,' she said.

We walked home, stopping off at the corner store to buy a bottle of Lucozade. According to the label Beecham Bros supplied this energising drink by appointment to HM the Queen, which Juan imagined she probably swigged in large quantities to fortify her in her battles with Mrs Thatcher. He was becoming increasingly preoccupied with food. Between the consoling visits to Dr Wall there had to be something he could do to arrest the loss of weight, to take control of this thing, to ward off the fear. For a couple of weeks he consumed prodigious quantities of carrot and celery juice. Then he heard from a friend that a watercress diet might be beneficial for his stomach. Fortunately the first bunch we bought at the market was so full of grit that he rapidly decided there was more to be said for another suggestion: a massive intake of cruciferous vegetables.

Unconvinced by these dietary experiments, I was grateful when Ann in her practical way produced a more promising alternative, a cookbook called *The Taste of Life* based loosely on the Pritikin diet to which the author had been converted when her husband had been diagnosed with cancer.

Juan went through the book methodically ticking approved recipes: corn fritters; chicken chow mein; fish in mango sauce; *kokanda*, an African fish dish with bananas and chilli and lime juice. All of this was perfectly in character. Astonishingly, though, he also ticked his way thickly through the pasta section. How many times had I listened to his set piece—in restaurants, at dinner parties, in the supermarket—about the nauseating smell of boiled pasta that conjured up the rationed poverty of his childhood? For all my attempts to cajole and persuade him, he had remained rigidly, monumentally opposed to eating pasta. And now, without comment, he suddenly relented, though he had the presence of mind to underline one sentence in the introduction for my benefit: '*A gradual change in diet is recommended.* This will allow your digestive system to appreciate the changeover without too much wind.'

Sadly, *The Taste of Life* was no more successful in settling his stomach or arresting the weight loss than my own improvised recipes. And the sense of crisis heightened when, despite the evidence of the billabong drawing, eating became painful for him. Simply swallowing a full meal was now an achievement, followed, as often as not, by the disappointment of regurgitating it a few minutes later. Night after night we sat down to dinner, our one firm, unalterable ritual of normality, and ended with a plate of vomited food and tears. 'Try smaller meals more frequently,' the hospital dietician advised. 'Six times a day.' By now it was early November; the teaching year at the University was mercifully finished and I sat at the kitchen table with bundles of exam essays, obsessed with food and dividing my attention unequally between lentil soup and the rise of fascism. Six times a day.

Sitting on the carpet in front of the gas fire he regularly monitored the changes in his body. On the lower part of his legs the skin had begun to flake and he rubbed them with coconut oil the way Indian mothers rub their babies. At the back of his legs where the calf muscles ought to have been there was an ache. He would pull up his tracksuit bottoms and take off his ski socks and say, 'Give me a treatment, Johnny.' And then, because his back ached as well, one day he stripped off entirely and lay face down on the carpet for what he called a full treatment.

It was odd, as I suddenly realised, that I had not seen him naked for some weeks. In using the bathroom he had always been very private; in bed he had taken to sleeping almost fully clothed. But here, stretched out on the carpet where the coffee stains were, there was no concealing his wasted condition. I was shocked; shocked by my own blindness; shocked by the weeping red eye of his *culi*, as he affectionately called his arse; stunned by the loose dark Buchenwald folds of skin that were all that was left of his buttocks. Searching for words, I found none. I said nothing, just as I had said nothing when he told me he could no longer get an erection. But he seemed not to expect words. He simply took my hands and guided them, as if I were a blind man, to the points on his spine and shoulders and his neck where I could knead away the pain.

He knew better than I did when it was unnecessary to speak. He also knew, more freely and fantastically than I did, how to dream and, in a fitful kind of way, how to hope. We were hearing reports of AZT, a new drug that was being trialled in the States, and these refocussed this thoughts on America, regenerating in him the old illusion that if only he were in a different place he might somehow discover himself to be a different person. In America he had not been sick, or at least not sick like he was now; and if they were going to discover a cure, a wonder drug that would knock out this virus, surely it would come from there. He believed, he very much wanted to believe in America.

Yet America had not saved Rock Hudson. It did nothing for the desperate men from Los Angeles who were running the drug trail to Mexico in search of a miracle cure. AZT sounded more promising than the do-it-yourself cures of the AIDS underground; but the more he thought about it,

136

the more both AZT and America itself receded into an un-attainable dream. Everything about the idea of returning was hopeless. We could hardly afford the airfare, let alone the obscene price that Burroughs Wellcome found it proper to charge for their new drug. And even if we made it to New York, there was no apartment, no family, no medical insurance to come home to. At the end of the road there would be at best a public hospice. That prospect shattered the fantasy. In his battle with New York City, beginning with those immigrant days in Hell's Kitchen, Juan had come out on top, and he wasn't about to let it claim him as a victim now. He did not want to die, he told me, like a common faggot.

'To die': the words slipped out more as a rhetorical flour-ish than a statement of personal fate, as though dying were a condition that applied in the streets and hospital wards of New York, on the other side of the world. Nevertheless, in those weeks when the gas fire was still burning late into the spring, it was evident that he was circling around the notion of death, brooding over it, hardly daring to name it. It was on his mind the night when he slipped back into bed after a trip to the bathroom and I felt him sobbing. 'I'm so frightened,' he said, and that was all. It surfaced on the night when we farewelled Paul and Tim, two friends who were leaving on a European holiday and spending Christmas at Santiago de Compostella. 'Yes,' he said brightly, 'I would like one day to go to Compostella,' and then a cloud passed over his face, which they remembered when they came to the place and lit a candle in the cathedral there.

Most memorable was the night of the Thanksgiving dinner. In the normal course of events Thanksgiving would have slipped by in our corner of the world unremarked and unobserved, someone else's festival. But when that some-one else was Juan, it was an occasion that demanded to be celebrated. So the cast of the birthday party was reassembled, minus the bishop and his wife, and we moved the venue next door to the priest's dining-room which could more easily accommodate the crowd. A 1959 edition of the *Better Homes and Gardens Holiday Cook Book*, a ten-cent bargain that Juan had picked up at a University book fair, provided the recipes and ritual rules. The book told us we should remember to be grateful for our liberty, which sounded reasonable, but it made no mention of speeches or toasts. Did one make speeches at Thanksgiving? Juan obviously thought so. At the end of the meal he was on his feet at the head of the table, composed, unusually quiet in himself and wanting to speak. He wished to thank Father Jim and Ann for their hospitality; he was glad that we had come as his guests. He knew that there were some of us who didn't think much of America and he wasn't going to argue about that. He wanted only to say that for him this was a special occasion.

'It's my last Thanksgiving.' There was a pause and then, as though he were shocked at the import of his words and their frankness, he added, 'I mean, as an American.' He asked us to fill our glasses for a toast, and in the moment all the million things that are America contracted to the span of Juan G. Céspedes.

'To America!' he said, and we drank to him.

Last celebrations, last performances, last things. This was one way of imagining the possibility of dying. Of course this quality of lastness was not always as sharp, as definitive, as easily recognised as that Thanksgiving. Sometimes—it must have been like this with his erections—there was simply no last to remember, only the dull sense that there must have been a last because there would be no more. But most certainly there was a last dance. It was on the night after Thanksgiving in the parish hall. Why the parish was having a dance I no longer remember. Perhaps they were raising funds, as they usually were, to repair the bits of the church that were continually crumbling and falling down; or perhaps, because it was spring, they simply wanted to dance. And so did Juan.

We arrived late. He was always late, but apart from that, it took him longer to prepare himself now, longer to arrange his ringlets so that the thinness would not show through, longer to re-iron the shirt that I had ironed too haphazardly for his fastidious taste. He tucked the shirt and two pullovers into the top of his leather pants, and then, going to the wardrobe, he took out the fur coat that had hung untouched throughout the winter and draped it extravagantly over his shoulders. He considered the effect in the mirror, and then, as a final touch, he put on a pair of reflecting sunglasses that had been *de rigueur* in the butchest heyday of Christopher Street. He was ready for the ball.

For much of the evening he sat at one of the tables arranged around the edge of the dance floor, chatting and accepting the attention of friends and well-wishers like the celebrity he undoubtedly was. When he danced, swaying slowly so that the coat rippled around him, it was with a Peruvian woman he had met at Mass the previous Sunday. She was a nervous, bird-like creature, more Indian-looking than Spanish, with a waif of a daughter called Delicia and a drunken Australian husband who had brought her back like a souvenir from a South American tour. The marriage was less than satisfactory, and as she spoke no English and the husband spoke no Spanish, the means for resolving their matrimonial difficulties were severely restricted. All of this, it appears, she confided to Juan as she danced and nuzzled her face from time to time into the fur of his coat. He was speaking in Spanish, for the first time—as far as I knew —since he had left New York. Later in the evening he approached the husband.

'You must look after your wife and the little girl,' he said. 'And you must stop drinking.' The man was too drunk or too surprised to take offence. Whether he stopped drinking, I never heard, but in due course Juan was pleased to hear from Father Jim that the woman and child had been returned, as they wished, to their native land.

That was the last time Juan danced. He was a star that night, and he shone more brightly because his sickness was so evident. He no longer attempted to mask it, but drew attention to himself as if to say, 'This is my coming out.' People asked each other, 'Is it cancer?' They asked me, 'Is it terminal?' They couldn't quite bring themselves to say, 'Is it AIDS?' They had never seen AIDS. No one in our circle had seen it. Only Juan, who had nursed Jerry on his death-bed.

*

It is sometimes said, and as frequently denied, that suffering can be ennobling. I don't think it ennobled Juan. What it did, though, was induce in him a fuller acceptance of that responsibility for himself that he had so long resisted. He made decisions; and, as far as it was possible, he took charge of his own fate. He wanted to find an alternative doctor. Not that he had any reservations about Dr Wall, nor any principled objection to orthodox medicine. But the intervals between the three-weekly appointments with Dr Wall at the hospital were becoming too long and, inevitably in a public hospital, the consultations, though they were never hurried, always seemed too short.

So we found an alternative doctor, who, we were told, conducted his practice as though it were a form of meditation. He had grown up in the East and so it seemed unsurprising when we arrived at his house to find that his garden tinkled with chimes like a Buddhist temple. From the entrance hall we caught a glimpse of his living-room, an Aladdin's cave of silks and batiks and oriental lace artfully draped and piled high on tables and flung nonchalantly over the chairs. Out of this cave emerged a woman with white skin and black eyes who guided us with a gesture of her bejewelled hand toward the surgery and into the presence of the alternative doctor.

Where Dr Wall was jovial and chatty as far as the situation would decently allow, this doctor approached his craft and his patients with a kind of mystical reverence. In the dim light of the surgery he moved silently, he wrote his prescriptions in silence, and when he spoke, the sound of his voice seemed rather to enlarge the silence than to diminish it. On Juan the impact of this cloistral atmosphere was immediate and, ever-sensitive to the ambience of his surroundings, he responded to the doctor with a soft passivity. For each suggestion of the doctor he was grateful. Yes, he agreed that it would help if he were to sit each day in a beautiful place, a garden for example, and open his mind to the influence of its serenity. Certainly he would practise the doctor's suggestion and try by the exercise of his will to hold his bowels a few seconds longer. And of course he would take the vitamin supplements that the doctor recommended.

Whatever the power of positive thinking, and however great the restorative powers of nature might be, Juan's belief in them evaporated rapidly when we left the surgery.

As far as he was concerned, the most beautiful place to sit was where his *culi* was not sore and his back would not ache. That place was the second-hand armchair that he had bought on a shopping expedition with Murray. It was massive and ugly, but you could pad it with pillows and you could snuggle into it in front of the TV and enjoy the beauties of nature—he liked watching Jacques Cousteau—in something approximating comfort.

The pain in his back grew more acute, and in his neck as well. He determined to consult a chiropractor. He chose a name almost at random from the yellow pages. It was a name of which the owner was evidently extremely proud, for when we entered his premises we were confronted with the name again, framed in gold and displayed prominently in the reception room, where it seemed to confer a special prestige on the Californian institution which attested to the doctor's manipulative skills. But more than the large ego and the trans-Pacific credentials, it was the snakes, or rather the wall-charts with their snakish representations of human spines, that prompted in me a wary reserve. And what was one to make of the slogan that announced: 'The spine is the human switchboard controlling health and vigour'?

I was glad that Juan took charge. After briefly indicating the nature of his problems to the doctor, he raised the question of the fee and began to haggle about the price as though he were dealing with a New York street vendor or a cut-price electrical goods store. Chiropractors—or their patients—were not covered by Medicare, and so the fifty per cent discount that Juan negotiated meant big savings. And in retrospect the half-price deal that he secured seemed well-justified: the pain in the neck went away but the back, said the doctor, would require a more extended treatment.

After the initial visit I was pleased to be excused from further attendance, something that never happened with a real doctor. But this was after all more like visiting a gym than a surgery, and for Juan it felt more like home ground. Even so, it was humiliating, painful to bare his body, so pathetically thin, and to measure it against the husky muscularity of the snakeman. Of the reason for his frailty, he said nothing.

Twice a week at 11.30 he went for this treatment. Then, with the old careful planning of his day that I remembered from his student days in New York, he would walk to a Chinese cafe in the city where you could buy a plate of barbecue pork and rice for a couple of dollars. From there he went on round the block to the State Library, taking the lift to the newspaper room on the second floor. He wanted to help me complete some research I was doing on colonial gardens. For two hours, or as long as his bowels permitted, he would work through the microfilm reels of nineteenth-century papers, indexing the articles in the gardening columns. He would have stayed longer, but the springs in the clapped-out seats pressed intolerably into his buttocks so he had to stand, stopped over the microfilm readers until his back could take no more. Those afternoons, and that pain, were a present to me. The entries in his spiral notebook finished abruptly with 9 September 1871: 'The Function of Melbourne's Botanic Gardens.' It was then that he lost control of his bowels and the mess ran down the inside of his legs and seeped through the seat of his cotton pants. He cleaned himself up in the lavatory where nobody could see his tears.

That was in mid-January. The diarrhoea was becoming more virulent. Each meal demanded a new effort of will and brought a new disappointment when it ended in a pool of vomit. His weight was still falling. How long could this go on? If his muscles were dissolved and his skin shrunken and stretched on the bones, how much more weight could he lose?

They were restless nights that January. Mostly he made it to the bathroom in time, but sometimes there was no warning. A change of sheets, a fresh diaper; everything seemed to proceed in slow motion in the yellow night light, and then we would settle again. I wanted to hold him, but he grumbled that my arm across his back was too heavy to bear. When I turned over to my side of the bed so that we lay back to back, he took it as a rebuff. Or worse. 'Are you afraid to hold me?' he asked.

He dreamed. One night his grandmother came to him and offered him a mango from the tree in her yard, but when he bit into it, peeling back the smooth skin with his teeth, the flesh was a mass of worms.

All that month Dr Wall was away on holidays. We received no joy from the young doctor who stood in for him at the clinic. He routinely renewed the prescriptions for Zantac and Imodium as though he were prescribing pills for a headache. But what about the loss of weight? Didn't he see that this couldn't go on? Didn't he recognise an emergency when he saw one? Well, perhaps he did: but Dr Wall would be back in a couple of weeks and this was his responsibility.

I phoned the alternative doctor and we took a cab across to the tinkling garden. The doctor went through his usual motions and looked grave and sat down at his desk on the far side of the room near the leaded window. Still lying on the couch where he had been examined, Juan raised himself on one elbow. It was time for the evasions, the kindnesses, the determined optimism to come to an end.

'Do I'm dying, doctor?' he asked.

The doctor had not been listening. 'I'm sorry, Juan, what was that?'

He repeated the question, his voice thick and low. 'Do I'm dying?'

Perhaps it was the curious trick of his syntax that distracted the doctor. 'I'm sorry,' he said. 'I didn't catch what you said.'

And so for a third time he asked. 'Do I'm dying?' The words hung in the air, no more than a whisper.

The reply was slow in coming. Then, simply, 'I don't know Juan. I don't know.'

That was the last time we saw the alternative doctor.

CHAPTER NINE

As the greatest misery is sickness, so the greatest misery of sickness is solitude.

—John Donne, 'Devotions'

Writing out yet another prescription for the hospital pharmacy, Dr Wall was evidently debating with himself.

'On second thoughts,' he said, 'perhaps you should come in so we can do a thorough check.' On our side of the desk Juan's hand searched for mine. Relief mingled with fear. 'Coming in' meant that we had reached the next stage of the sickness. Yet the doctor talked cautiously, and there were still few signs of that fatal blossoming that clinicians defined as full-blown AIDS, as though the disease were some dark rose with a terrible perfection of its own. Before that appalling ripeness was achieved there was a stage, it was said, that was diagnosed as ARC: and if one had to label it, this was now Juan's condition. In this evolutionary view of the disease there was still time. That was a comfort. And Dr Wall's decision was, after all, only a *second* thought, and the prospect of a stay in hospital, or indeed of any decisive intervention, relieved the helplessness we both had felt in that long summer.

Going to hospital is like preparing for a long journey, only more solemn. On the Saturday morning before he was due to be admitted, Juan packed his airline travelling bag and despatched me on a shopping trip to the city with a precise list: slippers, four pairs of thick ski socks, three fleecy tracksuits in bright colours in lieu of the odd assortment of singlets and pullovers he normally wore in bed, and a dressing-gown—or rather, in his words, a bath-robe. The bath-robe gave his preparations a certain grandeur. He had never possessed one. They had not been regarded as a high priority in revolutionary Cuba, and even in bourgeois societies there were a hundred and one more economical ways of keeping warm between the bed and the bathroom. But if you went to hospital, he imagined, there were certain proprieties to be observed and minimal standards of elegance to be maintained. Happily, he was delighted with the white Italian creation I brought back from Myer's; so pleased, in fact, that he offered to make a similar one for me. 'When I come home,' he said.

They had promised to call us some time during the weekend, as soon as a bed became available. By Sunday afternoon we had still not heard. I rang the hospital and was answered by a Prussian voice which said that it had no idea what I was talking about.

'Please do not waste my time,' it barked, managing to imply that I was a nuisance caller who specialised in harassing medical angels. 'You do not appear to realise that I have some very sick patients to attend to.' Well, I replied, I was very sorry (though not surprised) that his patients were so sick, but I also had a sick and very anxious patient who was waiting to come in. 'I know nothing about it,' said the Prussian angel, and hung up.

Half an hour later a call to the registrar produced a more helpful response. Yes, there was a bed available and Juan should come in when he was ready. The Prussian, who was only a resident, had been ill-informed. Still musing over this unexpected introduction to the arcane hierarchies of the hospital world, we walked down the street in the early evening, and Juan delivered himself as instructed to the care of the charge nurse on Ward 3 North.

When I arrived at the appointed visiting hour the next afternoon, he was asleep: sedated, I supposed, after the investigation. Slipping into the vinyl chair by the bed, I leafed through the Penguin copy of Thomas Mann's letters that I had been reading, trying to remember where I had left off. A 1920 reference to *Death in Venice* caught my attention. The subject of that story, Mann explained to his correspondent, was 'passion as confusion and as a stripping of dignity—what I originally wanted to deal with was not anything homoerotic at all'. Nevertheless, he had no objection to 'that emotional tendency'. He did indeed draw the line at 'repulsively pathological elements' which 'may be and frequently are involved'. But when he contemplated the examples of Michelangelo and Frederick the Great and Stefan George, he concluded that there was a 'good deal of high humanity in the tenderness of mature masculinity for lovelier and frailer masculinity'. Where, I wondered, would I fit into Thomas Mann's scale of disembodied, sexless manhood? Repulsively pathological? Tenderly mature? And what about that frailer and lovelier piece of masculinity that was still asleep in its canary-yellow tracksuit on the bed beside me? Did frailty exclude maturity? For all his liberal

148

instincts, Thomas Mann on homosexuality, I decided, was a sentimental ass. It occurred to me that he would have found the subject of AIDS irresistible: pathology, passion and youthful death. Savagely and unreasonably, I was glad he was not around to write about it.

Absent-mindedly, I left the book on the bedside table. It was still there in the morning when the ward inspection took place. In ward time, this inspection was the ceremonial high point of the day. Somewhere around mid-morning a procession of doctors formed. Moving from bed to bed, they drew the curtains around their solemn deliberation and then, like priests emerging from the sanctuary, they reappeared, always observing the same order. First came the director of gastro-enterology, reserved, formal, moving with all the *gravitas* that befits the head of a distinguished department. Black, polished shoes, I noticed. Next came Dr Wall, in brown suede. Behind him came the registrar, with blond curls and Scotch College good looks that Juan found decidedly sexy. Then, bringing up the rear, came the Prussian.

It was not usual for visitors to penetrate the sanctum behind the drawn curtains, but I was there anyway. Not much was said. They were waiting on the results of yesterday's tests. But the Prussian who was only a resident had to be put through his paces. Juan met his clinical questions with a brevity that might have been interpreted as surliness, and his voice sounded slightly slurred. The Prussian, who had probably boned up on AIDS overnight in the latest textbook, must have suspected a neurological disorder. Getting nowhere with Juan, he turned to me.

'Is he always speaking like this?' Then, without waiting for an answer, his eye fell on the copy of Thomas Mann's letters.

'Ah,' he said, 'Thomas Mann. He is one of our greatest poets. A difficult writer. If he is reading Thomas Mann, then there is no problem.'

The director's face remained impassive, and there was no way of knowing how he assessed the literary diagnosis of his resident. But the registrar gave a sexily subversive shrug of his shoulders. And Juan, half turning away from the phalanx of medicos, gave me a long slow wink that broke into a mischievous smile.

By late afternoon when I returned, he was alert and taking a lively interest in the comings and goings on the ward. The bed in the far corner was now vacant. In the next bed by the door was a businessman with a jaundiced face and a horribly distended stomach. Mid-fifties, Juan reckoned. A trio of junior executives appeared and grouped themselves uneasily around his bed, surreptitiously glancing at their watches, evidently more at home with their office routine than with the embarrassing duty of consoling a dying boss. Mostly his wife sat beside him, expensively silver-haired and navy-suited. Once she spoke to me while we waited for the lift.

'Your friend looks very ill,' she said. 'So young.'

Two days later when they took her husband away and she came to collect his things, she sat for a while with Juan.

'May I give you a goodbye kiss?' she asked, with that impulsive kindness that grief can release. She kissed him on the forehead.

'Thank you, my dear,' he replied.

The fourth bed was occupied by a modest little man to whom fate, or some youthful vulnerability, had attached a thoroughly immodest wife. From her ample exposure in the media I recognised her at once. She was, in fact, a Dame

Commander of the British Empire, and such was her capacity to command, it seemed a shame there was so little Empire left to benefit from her talents. From her post by her husband's bed she issued one salvo of orders after another, more or less indiscriminately, at anyone who strayed into her field of fire. She had begun her distinguished career as a nurse, and in her day they would not have tolerated the slovenly and unprofessional behaviour she encountered in the girls in this hospital.

'To think', she said, 'that this place once had a reputation. It's a disgrace.'

She glared at Juan, not from any particular concern for him but because that seemed to be the way she regarded the world in general. 'An absolute disgrace,' she repeated, demanding the confirmation which Juan obligingly supplied.

'I think so too,' he said.

'Yes,' she continued, whooping with indignation, 'and they pay my husband no attention whatsoever.' (Which, I thought, might well have been a relief for the poor man.) 'He had a hypo in the night and they phoned me at two in the morning and I had to come in all the way from the suburbs and the taxi fare was twenty dollars.'

In view of his alleged neglect, the little man's recovery was not far short of miraculous. On the third day of Juan's stay he was almost ready to leave. But first he would need to be spruced up, said the Dame, who sailed in with her personal hairdresser in tow.

'I've brought Kevin in,' she announced, as though she were introducing a pet parrot. We watched while Kevin set up an improvised salon by the little man's bed, flouncing and snipping with exaggerated artistry.

'Such a queen!' said Juan, in a tone that was intended as an aside to me. Instead, his comment carried around the ward. The Dame looked daggers, but Kevin enjoyed the attention and cocked his little finger more archly by way of acknowledgment.

Next it was Juan's turn to move. However diverting the society of the ward may have been, occasionally the lack of privacy was also distressing. Twice he missed the emergency pan beside the bed, which left a puddle of reddish diarrhoea on the floor. Apart from the stench, the nurses were worried about the risk of infection, and when the opportunity arose they moved him to a single room on 5 North, a light, white room with a large window that looked west over a single claret ash by the wall of the hospital chapel. It had been a cool, moist summer and the ash, I noticed, was still a lustrous green that was unusual for that time of the year.

Juan was the first AIDS—or ARC—patient on the ward, and one of the first in the whole hospital. That, and his Peter Pan youthfulness, gave him a special status. 'And those baby eyes,' Arlene remembered. Arlene was the charge nurse, genially bossy but anxious too, like most of the nurses, about how she and her team would cope with nursing an AIDS patient. 'We were a bit irrational for a while in handling it,' she told me later. 'Afraid. Afraid of not knowing.'

Quite apart from the virus, for some of the nurses I was a problem too, as I realised when I encountered one of the students at the corner store.

'Are you finding it difficult?' I asked.

'Oh no,' she said, 'of course we have to take special pre-cautions, but it's not too bad.' She paused and blushed. 'I don't think there's anything wrong with being homosexual,' she said. 'It's just that, well, I never really knew one before.'

That their nursing betrayed no sign of their apprehension was due in no small measure to Val. In her capacity as the infection control officer, Val ranged freely through the hospital sniffing out golden staph, inspecting nurses' fingernails, radiating commonsense and now calming the fear of AIDS. The fear was worst with the food assistants. They may not have seen the sign attached to the head of the bed on which was written in black letters: BLOOD PRECAUTIONS. But they certainly knew the gossip, and it was confirmed by the tell-tale signs of the red plastic bags near the door, bags that contained infectious, high-risk soiled lined. And so, until Val intervened, they dumped his dinner on a table outside the door and left it to go cold.

Juan was outraged. It was not that he wanted their bland food. In fact, after the first week he refused to touch it and preferred instead that I should prepare his meals and bring them in and eat with him. Was this OK with the staff? I enquired. 'Certainly,' they said. 'Lots of patients with ethnic food requirements do that.' Ethnic? I was startled to hear it said so matter-of-factly that our food was ethnic, though I could see what they meant. We *were* different.

The food assistants learned. In the evenings there was even one who called Juan 'possum' and brought the coffee and cakes to his bed with an extra cup for me, which was strictly against the rules. But the TV man, from whom we hired a set for fifteen dollars a week, was incorrigible. Juan kept a twenty-dollar note ready for him in the top drawer of his bed-table, but the man would not enter the room, relying on me to pay him at the door. He was the living embodiment of Juan's recurring nightmare of isolation, of detachment from human society, and he had to be dealt with.

'*Make* him come in, Johnny,' Juan pleaded. So with the

bed between me and the door I would hold out the money like a morsel of fish to entice a frightened cat. And like a frightened cat he edged forward and snatched it, retreating to the safe distance of the doorway to produce the five dollars change which he left on a convenient chair.

Within a few days the room began to assume a homelier, lived-in look. The TV reproduced the familiar sights and sounds of our domestic evenings: the six o'clock news, *Sale of the Century*, *The Colbys* and *Dynasty*, *Dallas* and the pre-season football. Val produced a poster of a super-athletic Nureyev in full flight which we blu-tacked on the wall. Paul and Tim, just back from their Spanish expedition, brought a tiny pilgrim statue from Compostella which shared pride of place on the bed-table with Juan's own album of studio photos. He had asked me to bring them in to show Arlene and Val, for though he would never say so in so many words, he wanted them to see how once his legs had danced, and how accomplished, how beautiful he once had been.

And there were flowers, from Rickard, and from the garden. Late summer flowers, worlds removed from the thripped-out, delicate, diaphanous things of spring, flowers that poured their energy into raw tough colour: zinnias and marigolds and 'Papa Meilland' roses charged with the warm concentrated perfume of the season. And from Murray, who had just begun to work with a city law firm and was enjoying the delight of having money to spend, there were gerberas from the best florists. Originally they came, I once observed, from South Africa, and yet they were so sunny— like Murray, Juan said—that it was unthinkable to be too political about them.

'Why should the whites have all the best flowers?' Juan said; so we appropriated them to ourselves—as blacks—and assigned to the whites by way of compensation the whole hideous tribe of the proteas.

At the end of the first week Dr Wall had good news to report. Standing with his back to the bank of flowers and beaming like Father Christmas surrounded by a halo of gerberas, he explained that they had identified the cause of the dysentery-like condition as shigella, which could be treated with antibiotics. It was a small victory, he cautioned, but nevertheless, a definite breakthrough. Victories had been hard to come by in the last few months, so this one called for a celebration. That evening, when Dr Wall looked in, he found us dining on lobster and champagne.

Trying to gauge the extent of this triumph, I looked up shigella in the medical library. It was 'a genus of entero-bacteriaceae of the family escherichea that invade intestinal epithalial cells and cause bacillary dysentery'. More interest-ingly, it was named for the Japanese bacteriologist Shiga who, I learned, had worked in Germany with Paul Ehrlich who was the uncle of Hans and Klaus of the Jewish textile family. Juan was pleased with this piece of information, as though it gave him an insider's advantage over the bacteria. In an odd way, it helped to be able to place them.

The antibiotics began to do their work, and the evidence was there in the daily record of his faeces: reddish, then less reddish, then brownish and less runny. The tendency was in the right direction, though the descriptions struck me as amateurish, unexpectedly impressionistic, compared with the usual scientific jargon of the doctors. Why didn't they adopt a standard colour code, or at least something more aesthetically pleasing, like the names in the box of Derwent pencils we had used as children: ochre, raw sienna, burnt umber?

The medical textbook included another, less welcome piece of information about shigella. In AIDS patients, it said, shigella was often resistant to therapy and tended to return after treatment. As Dr Wall had warned us, the improvement was only a *small* victory, a temporary respite. How long was temporary? And how energetically would Dr Shiga's bacteria reassert themselves? One question gave rise to another, obsessively. What about the weight loss? He was down now below forty kilograms. Would the antibiotics stop that? And what else could we expect? If this was not yet full-blown AIDS, what new horrors were lurking down the track? And how long would he have to stay in hospital, and how many bunches of gerberas would we need? And what if he came home in this weakened condition, barely able now to walk to the end of the corridor? The teaching year at the University was about to begin, and then how could I manage to be in two places at once? Compassionate leave? But did the University give leave to the partners of gay men, or was that something reserved for proper marriages? And the Immigration Department? What if they should now discover his condition and then, after twelve months of silence, decide that he was not eligible for permanent residence after all? The frenzy of questions exhausted me. I wished I could accept Dr Wall's advice, as Juan seemed to be doing, and take things step by step.

The daily routine of hospital life provided a buffer against these tormenting uncertainties, and within the institution we discovered moments that we could make entirely our own. Juan always had last use of the bathroom, another precautionary measure that had more to do with the shigella than with AIDS, and although he had to wait till mid-afternoon for his bath, he converted this necessity into a luxury.

By the time the room was free, the westering sun filled it with a tropical warmth that became infused with the scent of bath oils and the eucalyptus that he used in generous quantities. When I perched on the edge of the bath, shampooing his hair and soaping his back, there was nothing to disturb the simple pleasure of our intimacy.

One afternoon, when he sent me back to the ward for a box of tissues, I encountered the new senior resident in the corridor (the Prussian had been transferred). In our brief conversation the unstoppable questions welled up again. What might we expect? How long? And this time, shockingly, there was an answer.

'I'm afraid we have to face the fact that he is dying,' he said. Hesitantly, knowing he was taking a risk, he added: 'I'd be surprised if he had more than six weeks.' I collected the box of tissues and returned to the bathroom.

'Were you talking to the doctor?' Juan asked. Reluctantly, knowing that his hearing was very sharp, I said yes and resumed my position on the edge of the bath.

'What did he say?'

'Nothing much. I mean, he thinks they might have to do a few more tests.'

'What else did he say?'

'Well,' I said, stalling, wishing I had never asked for this information, 'he really didn't say anything.'

He persisted. 'Did he say I'm going to die?'

He had asked this question so often, though mostly of himself. He wanted to know, and there would be no easy way to tell him. I said, 'Yes.'

Without raising his eyes, he considered this for a while.

'How long?' he asked, in a strange flat voice.

Had he trusted me less, I would have lied, though my

evasion would never have stood the test of his scrutiny; but I was committed now, by all that our relationship had become. 'He said perhaps six weeks.'

With his head bowed over the water, he traced a circle with his index finger round a medallion of medicinal olive oil that was floating on the surface. In that moment there was just us; and the tap was dripping.

It was Juan who broke the silence. 'I'm getting cold,' he said, which was the signal to help him out and dry him.

The next morning he must have confronted Dr Wall with the opinion of the senior resident. He didn't mention it to me, and nor did Dr Wall, yet the slight reserve in the doctor's usually amiable manner seemed to indicate that he knew what had transpired, and disapproved. The senior resident should have kept his opinion to himself. As far as Dr Wall was concerned, we had certainly not reached the end of the road yet. With the shigella apparently under control, he wanted to tackle the gastritis or aesophagitis that made eating so nauseatingly difficult. The newly released drug, DHPG, that he wanted to use would have to be infused intravenously. In Juan's condition, he explained, that could more comfortably be done by using a porto-cath through which they could access a vein near the heart for the twice-daily hour-long infusions.

Implanting the porto-cath meant surgery. At Dr Wall's suggestion we went upstairs to talk with a woman who had lived with one of these devices for the past year. The sight of it was hardly reassuring. Juan stared at the plastic plug that seemed to have grown into her shrivelled chest. He had no questions, or at least none that he could articulate. If this thing was necessary, he would accept it.

They performed the operation, a relatively minor affair,

though the surgeon must have hated dealing with infected blood. There was a mishap. One of Juan's lungs collapsed, which raised the fear of pneumonia. They passed a tube into his chest to allow the air to be evacuated so that the lung could re-inflate. At the second attempt, they succeeded. Then the infusions began, with nurses gowned and masked, fearful of an infection that could spell disaster. When he bathed now, the porto-cath had to be protected with plastic and taped. The paraphernalia of sickness was proliferating around him.

Still there were worlds that remained intact and whole, places in his mind where the virus did not invade and disfigure and deform. One afternoon when he was hooked up to the drip, making a desultory attempt to concentrate on the pullover he was knitting, he announced a request.

'Johnny, I want you to buy me some *turrón*.'

'Some what?'

Out of his Cuban childhood the wish seemed so self-evident, so normal, that he flared up at my incomprehension and then, more patiently, attempted to explain.

'It's something you eat. There are two kinds: *turrón alicante* and *turrón jijona*. I want both. You can get it at the Case Ibérica in Fitzroy. They will have it there.'

It turned out to be a kind of nougat made with honey and ground almonds. When I brought it back in triumph, he made no attempt to eat it, but, insisting that I try it, he broke off a piece and popped it into my mouth like a communion bread. The remainder he put in the drawer of the bedside table where it went sticky, and we threw it out when he died.

Then, even more perplexingly, he wanted *caña*. Sugar cane. 'Of course,' I said, 'I'll see what I can do.' If he wanted sugar cane then somehow, by one means or another, he would have it, though where or how it could be procured in Melbourne I had no idea.

Walking down Collins Street later that day, impressed with the strangeness of the mission he had entrusted to me, I happened to pass the Queensland Government Tourist Office. On a hunch I went in. The receptionist was a study in hairspray and mascara. She sat at a desk in front of a large poster advertising the joys of the Sunshine State, a place, I recalled, where they had banned an HIV-infected three-year-old from her kindergarten and hunted her out of the country. When the receptionist wanted to know if she could help me, sir, I decided to waste no time with niceties. 'Yes,' I said, 'my lover is dying of AIDS and he needs some sugar cane to chew before he dies. Can you tell me where I can get some?'

'I'm afraid we don't have that kind of information,' she said. They wouldn't, I thought, but I tried again, making an effort to be more conciliatory. Surely she had some directories or address books, I suggested. They must be up to their necks in sugar cane in that part of the county, I reflected, and if you believed the papers they were certainly knee-deep in cane toads from Cape York to Brisbane, and what did cane toads have for breakfast if it wasn't sugar cane? But she was unyielding. Her business was holidays.

My business was finding sugar cane. At home I looked up the Yellow Pages and ran through the list of mills and refineries. They were no help at all, except, finally, for a suggestion that I might ask the people at the Queensland Department of Agriculture. They referred me in turn to a Sugar Research Institute in a place I had never heard of, and in this unknown dot on the cane-filled steppes—or whatever they are called in Queensland—I struck gold. They had twenty varieties under experimental cultivation, I was told, and did I have any specific requirements? A vision of the Berlin salami shop rose before my eyes, but resisting the temptation to panic, I replied, 'I'll leave that up to you. Just make it the sweetest and juiciest that you've got.'

'No worries,' said the man. 'We'll air-freight it down within the hour. Will five kilos be enough?'

At 7.30 next morning the parcel arrived with the cane neatly packed and wrapped in wax paper, and inside the box was a note that said, 'With our compliments and best wishes.' Queensland, it seemed, might even be worth a holiday.

Of all the changes and chances that accompanied his illness, none was more uncanny than the intervention of the African woman. With her husband and children she had been the previous occupant of our apartment. Juan had never met her, but when I saw her on the street outside the hospital one day, it occurred to me that she, who shared his tall lean blackness, might be a welcome visitor. 'Ward 5 North,' I told her. 'Come in any time after four.'

She had been, I explained to Juan, a refugee whom the parish had helped to resettle and support. What I did not know, but subsequently learned, was more important. When she had first left her native village for the big city, her mother had blessed her and told her that whatever else befell her in the city she should remember that she was an Anglican. Later, when her husband was out of the country and the city was convulsed with violence and she feared for her life and the safety of her children, the Lord Jesus wonderfully befriended and protected her. He opened her eyes, and she saw that her former devotion to Him had been mere lip-service. Really loving Him demanded something more.

As promised, she arrived at four. When she came in, Juan brightened perceptibly. She pulled a chair close to the bed and, after the briefest of pleasantries, she began.

'Juan, I want to bring you a message from the Lord.'

Suddenly there flashed into my mind the memory of a Baptist preacher who had once worked over my own dying mother. Sensing what was coming, I tried to head her off. We didn't need to talk about these things now, I said, but she would be pleased to know that Father Jim came every Sunday morning with the sacrament. Unfortunately, she didn't think much of Father Jim's religion. It was doubtful if he was saved, and anyway she wanted no truck with a veiled presence or wafers that were hardly even bread. What need of all of this when she knew the power of Jesus who could make her body leap and shake with faith and inflame her heart and speak His message on her ecstatic lips. If only Juan would talk to Jesus, really talk! It was hard working containing her, and I was grateful when another visitor came in and stopped the flow.

The Lord expects His friends to be resourceful, and in this respect the African woman was no slouch. When I arrived at my usual time the next afternoon, I found that she had been and gone already, and Juan was sobbing into the pillow. She had given him the full converting message.

'What did she say?'

'She told me about the devil, and hell.'

In my head I raged against the woman; I hated her; but my mouth stayed calm, and I heard it saying that I didn't believe in the devil and there was no need to listen to her crazy preaching.

'But my grandmother said the same,' he said, and I felt the shadow of Clara de la Rosa passing over us. 'If there is heaven, there is also hell. If there is God, there is also the devil.'

There was no profit in disputing with his grandmother. All I could do was sit on the bed and hold him.

'I'm so confused,' he sobbed. 'I don't know what to believe.'

With one arm around his waist to avoid the porto-cath and the drip, I just kept holding on. Later in the evening, when I was leaving, I pocketed the Gospel Ministry tape she had left and instructed the charge nurse *never, on no account, not ever* to let her back. And when I saw her husband, a genial, stately man of whom I was fond, I gave him the same message.

The sequel to this saga I heard from Father Jim. The next night he had a phone call from the husband to say that his wife was not well and the priest should come. Responding to this call, Jim hurried to the house where he found the woman lying on the bed in a trance, her eyes wide open, her hands moving rhythmically and her lips repeating a hypnotic chant. Having been prevented from returning to complete her work with Juan in the hospital, it seemed that here she was contending for his soul alone, and Father Jim would be her witness. She was locked in a mighty struggle with the powers of darkness, straining desperately toward a hard-won victory. But assuredly it *was* a victory.

'The Lion of Judah has prevailed by the Blood of the Lamb,' she exulted. 'He has trampled down Satan under His feet.' And so the battle chant continued until, in triumph, she announced the glorious news. 'Juan has been saved!'

After a few minutes another woman mysteriously appeared. Kneeling by the bed as the African thrashed and then subsided into a quiet exhaustion, she set up her own refrain, protecting her sister in her weakened state from the wiles of the devil.

'I bind you, Satan, by the Blood of the Lamb. You will not touch the servant of the Lord. Jesus, cover her with your wings. Wash her in your Blood. I bind you, Satan …' And so it continued.

In this unexpected way the process of Juan's salvation was accomplished, and when Satan was securely bound as well, the woman left as silently as she had come and went home, I suppose to wash the dishes. When the African woman had recovered and risen from her couch, it was time for Father Jim to leave too. Calling in at the hospital on his way home, he found Juan still wide awake, watching the TV, and Collingwood going down to yet another inglorious defeat in the night series.

It was several days before Juan reverted to the visit of the African woman. 'Why doesn't she come?' he wanted to know. 'She promised to come.' This time I *did* lie.

'Perhaps she has forgotten,' I said, and changed the subject.

While, unbeknown to Juan, the fate of his soul had been determined, the fate of his body was still under active consideration. Almost a year to the day since they had received his application, the Department of Immigration officials finally satisfied themselves that he met their requirements and sent a letter to that effect. Subject, of course, to a medical examination for which he should present himself, with the enclosed form, at the Department of Health. This was standard procedure, and in other circumstances we would have received the news with rapture. Now, on 17 March, 1987, it seemed like a cruel joke. Had he suffered from tuberculosis, epilepsy, convulsions or fits, from depression or high blood pressure? What was the state of his digestive tract, of his uro-genital system? Was he pregnant? Were there other abnormalities: hernias, varicosities or psycho-neuroses that might affect his ability to earn a living? There are times when it is better not to open mail, times when it is better not to know. I put the letter back in its envelope and wondered what to do.

After pondering the matter for the best part of a week, I phoned the immigration people and told them with reference to application V83/293 78 that Mr. Céspedes would not be able to keep their appointment because he was away from home for a while.

'Oh,' they said, 'where is he?'

I was tempted to tell them that he had gone to Ayers Rock for a holiday, but that would not have been helpful when they expected us to be at home together jointly paying the gas bills. So, with a desperate collapse of imagination, I said, 'Actually, he's in hospital, and he'll be in touch with you as soon as he comes home.'

'What's wrong with him?' they wanted to know, and I told them limply that I didn't know. 'I mean,' I said, 'I'm not quite sure. It's complicated. But we'll be in touch.'

When Juan asked, with one of those unpredictable rushes of anxiety, if the Immigration Department had been in touch, I said, 'No.'

I was disturbed by the decisions that the disease was forcing on me, uneasy with the interventions and subterfuges, the disclosures and withholdings that it seemed to make unavoidable. I was spending more and more of each day in the hospital, yet with each visit the established balance of our life together shifted, almost imperceptibly, but certainly.

Each step of mine into the outside world of work and mail and telephones, of connected activity, reinforced my sense of his captivity. Each night when I walked home with the dirty dishes—we always used the willow-pattern plates he had wanted as a Christmas present—I carried with me the guilty freedom of a deserter. 'Don't go yet, Johnny,' he would beg. The official visiting hours finished at eight, though after the first week we had never observed them. 'Stay till they bring the coffee.' 'Stay till the end of the programme.' 'Wait till the night nurse comes on.' Stay! Wait!

He had so much time in the hospital that he was beginning to lose track of it. 'How long have I been here?' he asked me one day. I couldn't remember exactly. It was certainly a long time, because all of a sudden his toenails needed clipping. And from the window I noticed that the claret ash had begun to turn, and a dark wine colour was seeping into the green. Six weeks, I calculated.

Apart from the drip and the complications of the porto-cath, there was no reason why he should not revisit the world. Indeed, he was hungry for it. He blazed with pleasure when Sebastian, the priest's son, invited him to a family dinner in honour of his eighteenth birthday. What kind of restaurant would he prefer? He chose Mexican. 'Do you remember?' he asked me. I did: the first time he had taken me to dinner in New York, at a Mexican taco bar where he knew the waiters and wanted to impress them with his friend from Australia. They had been, I recalled, obligingly complimentary.

By the usual standards of the restaurant-going public our evening as the guests of Carlos Murphy was undistinguished. Getting out of the car, Juan fiercely resisted my attempt to support him and stumbled over the bluestone cobbles in the gutter. We packed his chair with cushions and stared down the guests whose eyes kept darting at his gauntness. The tacos were soggy. The chilli had no bite. And he brought his dinner up anyway and we covered the mess on the plate with a paper napkin. We had coffee with Ann and Father Jim in their sitting-room, which was more comfortable, and as we were leaving Juan expressed his gratitude.

'Thank you, my dear,' he said to Ann. 'I didn't expect to see this room again.'

The night nurse welcomed him back. 'Did you have a good evening?'

'Great,' he said. 'Fantastic.' I undressed him and helped him into bed, and they came in with the drip which was several hours overdue.

Having regained a toehold in the outside world, he was eager to keep it, though he conceded now the need for a wheelchair. Whenever the weather permitted we went out in the afternoon, enjoying the dappled light under the elms in Royal Parade. From time to time he asked me to stop, to feel the breeze on his face, to watch a tram, to contemplate the students coming out from their classes in the Spanish mission-style conservatorium across the road. At the first corner we turned left by the high school to avoid crossing the gutter, then down the long row of poplars and beneath the high wall of the veterinary institute where he had wanted me to send the sick chooks. At the bottom of this path, where the pavement became rougher, he would invariably begin to protest, whether from the pain in his seat, or the fear of fouling himself, or the sheer cussed delight of asserting himself I could never decide. We covered the last stretch in a hurry. Safely back in the hospital foyer, taking care to avoid the Spanish-speaking woman at the reception desk, he would order a milkshake with a fine disregard for the inevitable consequences.

Then there was another opportunity for an outing. It was the day of the parish fete, a quaintly Edwardian occasion that has survived into the nuclear end of the century because people cannot resist a bargain or a pot of home-made jam. This year, unusually, it was being held in Lent, a breach of tradition that must have meant the parish was once again strapped for cash. In that case, it should have appreciated our custom, because Juan was in the mood to buy. After a couple of hours, which was as long as he could endure the discomfort of the wheelchair, we were back in the hospital with two dozen jars of preserves. For the nurses, he said, counting them off and matching them up with their jars: Lily, Angie, Lisa, Jackie, Bronwyn, Val, Arlene. Strawberry for Lily, he decided, because she was getting married, and marmalade for Angie because she was Scotch. And red plum for the one with the ruby lips.

He wasn't always so generous in distributing largesse. Occasionally he was vehemently, irrationally possessive. Like the time when Mario wandered into his room and helped himself to a fistful of plums from the basket of fruit on his table. It made no difference that Mario was demented and drifted around the hospital with a sign on the back of his pyjamas that said, 'If found, please return to Ward 5 North.' I heard Juan bellow from the end of the corridor, and by the time the nurse had removed the offending Mario and pointed him in another direction, Juan was in tears. 'He's stolen my plums,' he said, and the whole misery of his defencelessness flooded over him

Jam. Plums. Food. We were never far from the subject of food. Together, we still went through the morning ritual of ticking off choices on the hospital menu of lunches and dinners that he would not eat. Nor would he drink the Survimed, a complete food preparation that came like a soup-mix in little granules and two flavours, banana and oxtail. Out of deference to my efforts he would still struggle with some rice and chicken in the evening. Otherwise, by the time we entered the eighth week, he was surviving only on fruit. He had an insatiable desire for mangoes, the fat orange and green ones, until the season ended, and then the creamy-coloured thin ones that came with little gold stickers from the Philippines. And custard apples. When he first came in, he had been able to spit the pips across the room and hit the wall, and once he had scored a bull's eyes when he hit Nureyev in the crutch. Now he simply dribbled them on to a sheet of newspaper that I spread across the bed, and when he was finished I had to wipe the juice from his chin.

He was going down fast. Low thirties now. As the textbook had predicted, the shigella came back, and they started their colour count again. He was still on the drip, though whether it was doing any good, whether it had ever done any good, I never knew. The question was academic. He was dying.

There are books about death and dying. I hadn't read them. But I did have a vague sense that death was a process that one was supposed to talk about, to address, to work through. There were stages I was supposed to recognise and respond to. Yet since the day when I had broken the news in the bathroom, we had not mentioned the word. Juan alluded to it once or twice, indirectly.

'What will I do with my things?' he asked me one evening, and as so often the question seemed to surface out of nowhere.

'You'll have to think about that,' I replied, and my answer was swallowed up in his silence.

And then, most cruelly, in a way that I found unbearable, he was assaulted, battered with the idea of death. Not death in general, not as an abstract principle or a spiritual reality, but death as a victim of AIDS. In the weeks that he had been lying in hospital, Ms Ita Buttrose and her colleagues at the National Advisory Council on AIDS had been preparing a campaign to alert the general public to the gravity of the epidemic. There were 442 cases of AIDS in the country; 238 deaths were already recorded. They needed an approach that would shock, that would stop people in their tracks. 'We want to make it explicitly clear that AIDS has the potential to kill more Australians than World War Two,' Ms Buttrose announced. So they hired an advertising agency and unleashed the Grim Reaper on the television screens of the nation.

It would run for only two weeks, they said. But what comfort was that if they were the last two weeks you would spend on this earth; and when you were struggling to make sense of what was happening to you they confronted you with this fantastic cowled creature, socket-eyed and scythe-swinging, knocking down its victims like pins in a bowling alley? No mercy, was the message; violent, impersonal, death as a complete wipe-out.

The first time we saw it, I felt ambushed, stunned. The second time I got up to switch the channel, but Juan said, 'No, no. Leave it. It won't take long.' It was, after all, only the TV, and he hadn't spent all those hours, thousands of them, watching TV without knowing how it produced its effects. He knew that AIDS was not like that. And as for dying— well, we would see.

CHAPTER TEN

Enter with riches. Let your image wear
brocade of fantasy.

—Denise Levertov, 'To Death'

On the eighth day of the Grim Reaper, into the second week of the AIDS campaign, it was Palm Sunday. And the surprising fact was that the approach of this festival absorbed him more, far more than the neo-baroque chamber of horrors that Ms Buttrose and her team had sponsored on the TV screen. It is difficult to know what attracted him so powerfully to that day. It may have been the crowds, the crowds that would be in church, and the ancient crowds of Jerusalem, hosanna-ing and waving their palm branches, not so very different, perhaps from the crowds that Fidel had gathered in his wake when he swept into Havana, except that Fidel did not come on a donkey.

'You have been there, haven't you, Johnny?' he said, and I recalled for him again the memory of my visit to Israel, and how I had walked down the Mount of Olives and followed the procession of palms through the city gate and into the courtyard of the Latin Patriach.

'Tell Jim,' he said to me, 'that I will be in church for the palms.'

The measure of his eagerness was such that, when I arrived at the hospital that morning, he had long since been ready. He had organised the nurses to complete their work with the drip and to pack a day's supply of pills and boxes of Kleenex and an emergency bed-pan, and he had commandeered the best wheelchair on the ward and had it stationed by his bed overnight. While we waited for the car to collect us, I fetched a bowl of warm water and shaved him, holding his head steady with my left hand, and with the other trying to work the razor into the deep recesses of his cheeks. He subdued his impatience for a few moments and was pleased enough with my attempts, but his whole attention was directed toward the strenuous effort of the day ahead.

The ceremonies were already under way when we entered the church. The air was heavy with incense and singing; and behind and around the priests as they processed waved the palms—fan palms, wine palms, date palms and any other palms that could be procured for the occasion, stripped from gardens and purloined from railway sidings, decorated with roses and festooned with red and purple ribbons, palms sanctified now to the celebration of impending death. After the antiseptic whiteness of the hospital, the spectacle caught him up with peculiar force. As I wheeled him down the aisle beneath the arches of palms to a place at the front, he burst into tears, and hardly appeared to notice that there was a photographer present, and a reporter, as we learned later, from the *Times on Sunday*.

The Mass began. From the steps of the sanctuary they

solemnly narrated the gospel of the Passion from red books with gold crosses on the covers, and when they came to the end a small boy in the pew behind us said to his mother, 'What is wrong with that man?' 'He's very sick,' she replied, which apparently sufficed as an explanation.

Then they were praying: for the church, for the world, for the sick. The sick were surprisingly numerous. However, by virtue of their infirmity they were understandably absent, so that the roll-call of their names proceeded without interruption. But Juan Céspedes was there, and when his name was read, he responded quite audibly with a prayer of his own. 'Take away this pain,' he said; and if anyone glanced across at his wheelchair they would have seen that his head was bowed, as if in prayer, but equally because his neck could no longer hold it upright.

When the people had received communion and the priests were performing their concluding rites, there was a tap on my shoulder from the boy's mother. I turned around, and the boy passed across the pew a drawing of a man on a donkey and palm trees with blue fronds under an orange sun. 'It's for the sick man,' he said.

And the last hymn, with its confident, world-conquering Victorian piety, was that also for the sick man?

> *Ride on, ride on in majesty*
> *In lowly pomp ride on to die.*

I looked down at Juan. His feet had slipped off the footrest of the wheelchair and were splayed uncomfortably on the floor, but he was singing.

> *Bow thy meek head in mortal pain . . .*

So, with his palm cross tucked into the breast pocket of his white Italian dressing gown, he entered the holy week preceding the death of God.

Outside the church we were introduced to the reporter. He had been commissioned by his paper, which must already have been in a state of terminal decline, to write a feature article on 'What People Are Doing at Easter'. He needed to do some interviews, and our friend Judith, who could improvise a party out of thin air and a flagon of red wine, announced that he should do these over a lunch at her gallery. The photographer should come too. In fact, there was a more or less general invitation.

'You will come too, won't you, Juan?' And he said, 'Of course.'

It was in the gallery, in the midst of chatter about Easter and employment conditions at the *Times on Sunday* and the futility (or otherwise) of the peace march they would join in the afternoon and the necessity (or otherwise) of unilateral disarmament, it was here that Juan finally took his leave of Hiram. He had not been in touch with him for more than a year, and the remembrance of him now was prompted by the sight of a dish of pickled herrings.

'Jewish food,' he commented. 'Hiram eats these.'

And so, although he had always despised sour pickles, he asked for a piece of herring and nibbled it in a final communion with La Negra. But Jewish food no more agreed with his stomach than did Christian, and we had to stop the dog from licking up the pile of regurgitated fish on the floor.

The reporter made notes, which duly appeared in the paper at Easter, along with accounts from the Lakemba mosque and other centres of devotion across the country. At North Melbourne, the article said, they were high church without being high camp or highbrow. Father Brady, 'easy-going, slightly eccentric and politically left-wing', led an eccentric flock. This included the perennial Liberal candidate for the safe Labor seat of Melbourne, and Judith who ran the gallery, and a woman called Linda who would be camping in the bush with her family at Easter, 'making altars out of stumps and things like that'. And then there was Juan. 'Last Sunday, the friends of another member of the congregation, Juan Céspedes, were far less sure what he would be doing at Easter. They were not sure he would be alive. AIDS has ravaged his emaciated body and he can only attend church in a wheelchair.' It was accurate as far as it went, though I could never fathom why people were so impressed with the wheelchair. I wished they had written he was sick as a dog, but still elegant in his high-fashion bath-robe.

Early in the afternoon, when the luncheon party marched off with their peace palms, Juan and I came home. The cats poked their heads round the living-room door, a bit sniffily, I thought, for such a momentous occasion. I had put a vase of red gladdies on the table because he had told me once that these were his mother's favourite flower.

'My mother's favourite flower,' he said, acknowledging my gesture. Otherwise he was pleased to see that nothing in the apartment had changed in the nine weeks that he had been away. That was sufficient. He had seen enough and he was suddenly tired, anxious to return to the hospital. As we were leaving, and Ann and Jim came into the garden to farewell him, it occurred to me that we had forgotten the bag of pills that was still sitting unopened on the living-room table. Should I fetch them? 'No,' he said. 'I've taken enough pills. Throw them out.'

He was still asleep when I arrived on Monday morning with the bowl of strawberries that he wanted for his breakfast. The room looked different. Before I had left him the night before, he had asked me to take down the poster of Nureyev. When Val had brought it in as a present he had been delighted by her thoughtfulness. Now though, after weeks of gazing at that peerless athleticism, he found the image unbearable.

'Take him down,' he said. 'He's odious.'

The removal of Nureyev seemed to have been the signal for a wholesale reorganisation of the room. Some time during the night they had moved the bed, swinging it around by an angle of ninety degrees so that it faced towards the window and the western sun. Over the head of the bed, where it partly obscured the BLOOD PRECAUTIONS sign, one of the nurses had tied the palm cross which was bound with a bunch of French lavender he had been given at the gallery. It was as though they had set the stage for the final act.

Something about his sleeping disturbed me. He was definitely asleep: yet his eyes were half-open, but glazed, not seeing, and then he seemed to be speaking, or trying to speak, in a thick voice as though his mouth were nothing but tongue. And then, quite distinctly, I caught the word 'Mamá!'

Mamá! Was he back in Guantánamo, on the poor street where the long row of white houses closed their shutters against the summer heat? Or was he responding to those firece, embracing letters from his mother that he half feared to open, and that scorched and seared him with self-reproach and guilt? 'I hardly remember your face,' she had written, 'but I hope to embrace you before I die.' 'Write to me but

do not tell me lies. I want to know the truth of your life.'
'Do you still love me now that Rafael is big?'

Rafi! That was the second name he called out, brightly,
eagerly. Since he had heard that Rafi was in Germany, he
had hoped it might be possible to meet him there, in Berlin,
where he would cross through the Wall with a brand-new
American passport, thumbing his nose at the Communist
guards. And on the other side there would be Rafi, with his
muscles and his darker skin, so that you might have wondered whether they shared the same father. Or was it just that
Rafi looked more like his grandmother who was very black,
and who had long since gone to her rest and was buried in the
cemetery on the edge of the town where the *locas* used to
make out with their men, and where there were white marble
angels that had been erected before the Revolution.

Then he muttered a third name. 'María!' I was sure he
called María: but who was she? I ran through the list of
nurses in my mind. There was no María, but there was
Arlene, thank God, who now appeared with her usual cheerful bustle to assure me that, if he had not come round yet,
it was because he'd taken an extra sleeping pill.

It must have been an hour or so before there was any
further sign of life. Suddenly, very suddenly, his eyes shot
open with the startled-rabbit look that always made me
want to laugh.

'Am I dead?' he asked. It was not an unreasonable
question. After all, how should one know that one is dead
unless the death is certified? At the sound of my voice, he
was fully awake.

'Johnny!' he exclaimed, as though I was the last person
he might have expected to be at his bedside. 'Did you bring
the strawberries?'

Five days to Easter. What if he died at Easter, I wondered, on the longest of long weekends when even the corner milk-bars were closed and certainly, I presumed, the undertakers? What then happened to the dead? Were they lined up in a grisly holiday traffic jam, waiting their turn in an endless queue to enter their six feet of earth? The thought appalled me, and I determined that the funeral arrangements should not be left to chance.

At the edge of North Melbourne, where the distinct lines of the city merge into the amorphous expanse of the western suburbs, there was a firm of undertakers. They were, as I later discovered, the most expensive practitioners of their trade, and I reflected that Juan might well have disapproved my impulsive engagement of their services. He would have shopped around, found a bargain price, done a deal. But once I was through the smoked-glass doors and marching through the vestibule up to the reception desk, it seemed somehow indecent to calculate the cost.

'I would like to arrange for a funeral.'

The woman, who reminded me uncannily of the Queensland Tourist clerk, adjusted her spectacles and reached for a form.

'What is the name of the deceased?'

'Well,' I said, as the full enormity of this encounter hit me, 'actually there is no deceased.'

'Oh, I see, sir,' she said, 'I expect what you are referring to is a pre-paid funeral. Is it for yourself?'

That was certainly not what I meant. In fact, although I could not say as much to the receptionist, there was not enough money in the bank to pay for this one necessary funeral, let alone a pre-paid one for myself. I would have to apply for a loan, though as the bank was so keen to lend money for caravans and cars and holidays in Spain, I didn't anticipate any trouble in securing an advance for something infinitely more important.

Finally, when she understood the import of my visit, she summoned a grey man in a grey suit who escorted me into a counselling room. The neutral, understated, be-berbered look of this room aggravated me.

'I have to arrange the funeral of my friend,' I told the man, 'and I need to know if there are any special complications because of AIDS.'

He assured me that there were no problems.

'Is it true, though,' I persisted, 'that they put AIDS people in a plastic bag?'

'Well,' he replied, perfectly composed and with a fine evasiveness, 'the Health Department requires certain precautions in case of contagious diseases.'

I pondered this for a moment. Green plastic or black? At any rate, heavy-duty plastic, I supposed. Was this really necessary? I let the moment pass: it was not worth creating a fuss over a plastic bag.

We moved on to the details. To be burned or buried, he wanted to know.

'Buried,' I said. 'Definitely buried.'

'In that case, sir, we can offer you two options. All our work from this side of town goes to Fawkner or Altona.'

Of Fawkner I had no conception whatever. Altona, though, I knew from the window of the bus that takes you to the Public Records Office. A more dismal place would be hard to imagine; sprawled on the fringe of the western plains, littered with basalt boulders and Scotch thistles and enclosed with cyclone wire, it could hardly be distinguished from the chemical storage plants and transport depots that surrounded it. Even the gum trees there were stunted, twisted, buffeted by the unceasing wind.

'I'm sorry,' I said, 'they are both out of the question.'

He could see that I was going to be a difficult customer. Did I have any *particular* objection? It seemed unreasonable to tell him that the gates of the Altona Memorial Park, with their tacky iron lettering, reminded me eerily of Auschwitz. Instead, a phrase of Juan's sprang to my lips and I said quite simply, prim as a Toorak matron, 'They have no class.'

Such bare-faced snobbery startled the man, and he was so evidently pained that I was tempted to assure him that of course I knew he was not personally responsible for the miserable destination of his handiwork. As an alternative I suggested Kew, a nineteenth-century garden cemetery that had acquired with the passage of time an appealingly rural atmosphere. I had walked there as a child with my grandfather, hunting for lizards that sunned themselves on the tombstones and dropped their tails when you tried to catch them. The man was doubtful. There were plots available from time to time at Kew, but they tended to be in the rambling, unkempt end of the cemetery, where briar roses and kiss-me-quick ran riot over the graves.

That sounded perfect. Still the man hedged. They would need to dig the grave by hand, he observed, as though the reversion to this quaint practice of a bygone age offended his sense of advanced professionalism. As it had never occurred to me that they would dig the grave by any other means, that was hardly an objection. Kew would be ideal, I said, and a phone call confirmed the arrangement.

From the Counselling Room we moved to the Selection

Room, where the man brightened perceptibly in the congenial gloom. Here, it appeared, I would be required to choose between a casket and a coffin. He glided around the room, explaining the various shapes and timbers, lovingly running his hand along the polished grain of a deluxe model with satin padding. Moving down the scale, he advised delicately about prices, and as we left the caskets and entered the less ambitious coffin section, he confided to me supportively that there was after all something to be said for tradition.

What did I prefer? In fact, I found the whole extensive range repulsive. Yet in the few minutes of my acquaintance with the undertaking world, I had come to realise that it too had its pride, and if it had survived the assaults of Jessica Mitford and Evelyn Waugh there was no point in my tilting at it now. I side-stepped the question.

'Do you have nothing in plain wood' I asked. 'Pine, perhaps? Unvarnished, unpadded. I mean, more or less a box. Something natural?'

'No, sir,' he said. 'There is no demand for anything in that line.'

That being the case, it seemed best to settle for the simplest, least offensive coffin, a chipboard model with a dark veneer. 'A popular choice,' he told me, which I quite believed, as it happened also to be the cheapest. But the chrome-plated crucifix would have to go.

'Of course,' he said, 'that is for our Catholic clients. May I ask what is your religious affiliation?' My affiliation, I advised him, was C. of E., though what that had to do with arrangements for Juan was somewhat obscure. I thought I detected a hint of relief in his voice at this sign of normalcy.

'That will be no problem,' he said. 'For Protestants we

use a silver cross.' It seemed that everything they touched in this establishment turned to chrome. You couldn't win.

'I would prefer it', I said, 'if you would leave the coffin completely plain. No crosses, no crucifixes, nothing at all.'

'I understand,' he said, making a note in his book and, perhaps, a mental note as well: Lapsed.

That was all. Further details could wait till the time came. And I was anxious to get to the market before it closed, hoping to find there the guavas for which Juan had unexpectedly asked; the ones that were pink inside.

Wednesday

Improbably, as it seemed to me, on Wednesday he was still planning for the future. The previous Easter we had bought a marzipan lamb from Vito Barone's Sicilian pasticceria. Suddenly recalling this, Juan thought we should have another, and when I brought it in, he was freshly amused by its long neck and supercilious upturned nose, its tinsel halo, and its campy little legs with the painted toenails, delicately displayed on a ground of green jelly crystals. When Val dropped in to see how he was getting on, she admired the lamb.

'It's for Easter, Val,' he explained, and the words came out so slowly that it sounded like a most important pronouncement. 'Will you come to dinner with us at Easter?' She apologised that her mother would be coming to stay with her at Easter. 'Well, bring her too,' he said.

His anticipation of the forthcoming holiday was heightened by a visit later that afternoon from Alison, the bishop's daughter, who was flying in from New Zealand to help with the last minute preparations of a friend for an Easter wedding. When she came in with Ann direct from the airport, Juan greeted her with undisguised pleasure. It was almost nine months since her own wedding.

'I thought you would be having a baby by now,' he said. She laughed. Of all the visitors to the hospital, she was the most natural; and if she took in the drip and the bedpan and the rest of the paraphernalia of sickness, if she was startled by the skeletal frame that he had become, none of this affected the lively sympathy of her conversation.

How was the bishop? he enquired. The bishop was settled in retirement in a village in the Suffolk countryside. Did she remember the story about that other village, the place where the bishop had been sent as a young priest? It was a place so feudal that the cottagers depended for their electricity supply on a generator owned by the old woman who lived alone in the manor house. And she, to encourage habits of thrift and early rising, switched it off each evening at sunset, so that the bishop had to compose his youthful sermons by candle-light. So we reminisced and laughed our way through the bishop's stories until it was time for Alison to leave. Juan wanted to make her a present.

'I'll make you a linen suit,' he promised, 'with a silk lining.' And there would be one for Ann as well.

When they were gone, and I was sitting at the end of the bed massaging his feet, he asked, 'How much money is in my bank account?' In fact it was a joint account that we had opened, more for the sake of impressing the Immigration Department than for our own convenience. There was about a thousand dollars, or at least there would have been had I not been drawing on it to meet the incidental expenses of the hospital stay. He was disappointed that it wasn't more, but still, he hoped it would be enough.

'I want you to buy a carpet for the front room, and a washing machine,' he announced, 'a front-end loader.' For months we had been talking about the need for a washing machine. It wasn't easy to manage diarrhoea-stained sheets in the bath, and we didn't like to impose this kind of washing on Ann. We had decided that, if we could persuade the agent to pay for the plumbing, when he came home we would instal a machine in the kitchen beneath a bench near the sink. It would need to be a front-end loader. But why was he thinking now about washing machines?

The subject continued to preoccupy him, and he took it up with the social worker when she passed by on her round. We both felt sorry for the social worker. We liked her well enough, and she so much wanted to be useful. She knew of every pension entitlement and sickness benefit that the Department of Social Security had ever invented, and she had bunches of application forms, but there were no forms for a person in Juan's state of bureaucratic limbo—nor, for that matter, for his friend. Undeterred by her inability to assist us, she kept coming, in the manner of her profession ever hopeful, and now, after so many visits, came her moment. How much, Juan asked her, would a front-end loader cost? She didn't know exactly; she guessed around six hundred dollars. I watched his face as he struggled with this piece of information and calculated and came to the conclusion that, if this were true, there would not be enough left over for the carpet. He burst into tears and his head fell back and rolled sideways off the pile of pillows. A nurse who had overheard the conversation came to the rescue.

'Oh no,' she said, 'I'm sure you can get a washing machine more cheaply at a discount store.' This reassured him. She fluffed up the pillows and restored him to a more comfortable position.

'Why do you ask, Juan?'

'It's for the apartment,' he replied, close to tears again. 'For Johnny.'

This was his will, the first part of the answer to that question he had put to me some weeks ago. 'What will I do with my things?'

Thursday

The second part of his will he kept till the following evening. It was Holy Thursday, the commemoration of the Last Supper, the passover meal that ended at Gethsemane.

'Will you be going to Mass tonight?' Juan asked.

'No, I want to be here.' But perhaps in the night I would go to the vigil and keep watch for a while in the chapel of repose. If I could stay awake.

It was a long day, devoid of form, a mere prelude to the eventful evening. It was a day impregnated with the terrible sweet smell of shit. And he was sweating. And there was a last altercation with Angie, the Scotch nurse whose accent he loved, who was still valiantly trying to coax him into taking his pills. It was a contest of wills that she couldn't win. At his insistence, I had been throwing them into the bin all week.

He was waiting, waiting for Murray, who came in that evening as he had for so many evenings, to chat while we ate or to share our meal, to arrange his gerberas and remove the droopy ones, to punctuate the evening news with his irreverent comments. That night there was no news and no meal. The thermos flask of soup that I had brought at lunchtime was still unopened; it was still warm when I poured it down the hospital lavatory the next day.

He tried to keep up a brave front with Murray, but the tears kept breaking out. 'I'm dying, Murray,' he sobbed, 'I'm dying.' The storm passed, and when he was calmer he asserted himself with a great effort of will, and said very solemnly to Murray, 'I want you to have my bike, and my sewing machine.' The second part of his will.

The next visitor was Rickard, who had come with Ann from the evening Mass and was on his way to the airport to catch a plane to Dublin where he had to lecture the Irish on their contribution to Australian history. From there, when we telephoned him with the news, he wrote back, his memory still impressed with his last night visit to the ward: the strangeness, the eeriness of it and Juan, lying there, fearful yet oddly patient, the tiny tears finding their way down his cheeks.

Out of that patience came the greatest sadness, a sadness that lodged in me, it seems, for ever. Four short words, neither a moan nor a cry, but a simple clear statement of infinite regret. 'I have accomplished nothing,' he said. How formal it sounded, how hauntingly Latin in its choice of the word 'accomplished'.

They had always said that he wouldn't amount to much. Alicia Alonso said that when he wanted to dance for the National Ballet. It was the same with the professor at Marymount—what was her name?—Haila. Haila Schwartz had given him an F for modern dance, which he could hardly believe, and the only reason she gave was that she didn't like his attitude. Somehow it was always like that. Even when he played Lotto and tucked the tickets behind the icon of the Mother of Sorrows for luck, the numbers always fell the wrong way. Perhaps it would have been different if he had not left Cuba, if he had not set out that night with Alex through the salt flats. That had been a foolhardy thing to do when he couldn't swim.

He had accomplished nothing, nothing that people would remember, nothing that would cause them to honour in him the name that had been borne by Cuba's greatest patriot. He had not even finished his quilt, which still lay in a neat pile of patched squares on his sewing table.

There are poets who have written that death itself is a kind of accomplishment. Rainer Maria Rilke said something like that. 'O Lord, grant to each man his own death, a death that proceeds from his life.' That was all right for Rilke, with his pretty name and his faith in the great death that each one has within him. It was not what I wanted to say.

What I wanted to say to Juan had nothing to do with greatness. It was simply this: that he had loved me. But somehow it didn't come out like that. All I could manage, all I could give him, was the remembrance of our togetherness. 'There has been us,' I said. And I know that he understood, because somewhere in that night, in the fragments of his dying, he said, 'We made it, Johnny. Didn't we?'

The next time I looked at my watch it was nearly midnight. Rickard's plane would be departing. I sat on the bed, holding Juan's hand. He needed a haircut, I thought, and the long curls against his forehead were wet with sweat. He had made now, I supposed, all the decisions that had to be made, farewelled his friends, disposed of his things. And still he was waiting.

'Shall I call Father Jim?'

'If you like,' he said, as if it were I who needed to be supported for the rest of the way.

The priest came. 'I'm so frightened,' Juan confided to him, and I was taken aback by the marvellous matter-of-factness of Jim's reply.

'We'll see what we can do about that,' he said, in the drawling accent of his Botany boyhood. Priests deal in certainties, and this priest knew his craft. He slipped a stole around his neck, a strip of antique silk richly embroidered with gold.

'It's beautiful,' Juan said.

'You can hold it if you like.'

As he grasped the fringe of the embroidered stole, he noticed that further up it was fraying at the edges.

'I'll fix it for you, Jim,' he said. 'I'll need silk thread.'

There were prayers, and he was anointed on the forehead and again on the hands, and he received the sacrament that had been brought down specially from its lonely glory on the altar of repose.

We were very near the end now. He dirtied the bed, and when the nurses lifted him into the chair while they changed the linen, his eye fell again on the palm cross on the bedhead, and he instructed me to put it with him in his coffin. A second time his bowels moved. And then a third, and what came out looked like blood and water. Was it the guavas, I wondered?

Finally when he was quieter than he had been all day and appeared to be drifting off to sleep, I switched out the light.

'Come to bed, Johnny,' he whispered. So I took off my shoes and slipped into the bed beneath the blanket that was draped on a wire frame to spare his body the weight. I cradled him in the curve of my body and listened to his breathing. After a while I thought he was asleep, but he had one more question.

'What time is the vigil?'

The vigil? There were so many vigils in this religious season: the vigil of Holy Thursday, the vigil of Easter. And there was our vigil, which was all but over.

Good Friday

It was broad daylight when I awoke. The breakfast tray was on the bedside table. He was still asleep. I slid out of the bed, and walked home to have a shower and shave.

The phone rang. It was Arlene, who had just come on for the morning shift. Did I want to be there at the end?

I ran back, and waited. He didn't stir. Outside the window, I noticed, the claret ash had coloured magnificently. It had been a mistake to plant that crimson against a cream brick wall. The first leaves were dropping, floating really, early into the fall.

A nurse came in to sit with me. She brought a radio and switched it on to a programme of Easter music.

'Hearing is the last sense to go,' she said, and I marvelled at how much there was still to learn about death.

Bach. Rachmaninoff. Handel. A few bars into the Handel there was static on the radio, and I reached across to adjust the dial. When I turned back to Juan, he had died.

The news spread, and a small crowd gathered in the room by the time that Jim came to read the prayers for the dead. The palm cross was still tied with its ribbon to the bed. I thought about the heavy-duty plastic bag, and asked Arlene how we could be sure that he would have the cross in his coffin. Untying it, she placed it in his right hand, and clasped his fingers around it. The blood had drained from his face which was now a pale olive, and the African in him

189

seemed to give way to the Latin. He looked, I thought, like a Spanish nobleman.

A similar thought must have occurred to Ann.

'We should bury him in his fur,' she said. And so I came home to collect the fur coat and made my last trip, on his account, back to the hospital.

They had already removed his body.

CHAPTER ELEVEN

Let no one think,
because I am no longer crying…

—Humbert Wolfe, 'First Memory'

We buried him, as I had arranged, at Kew. On the high
ground, near the wall, in the shade of the pittosporums we
buried him with our own hands. As we brought the coffin
to the grave, some parish children followed the procession.
Nobody asked them to come, but they were there, as if to say
that death, this death, had touched us all. And so we committed his body to the earth from which it came. With rolled-
up sleeves, and sweating, we shovelled the yellow clay. 'You
can see who comes from peasant stock,' one of the women
said. And the gravedigger, who leaned against a fallen tombstone and watched from a respectful distance, told me that he
couldn't have done a better job himself.

It was more than a year before I was able to fulfil the
final obligation that Juan's death laid upon me. I flew to
New York, and then to Montreal to catch the weekly Cuban
Airways flight to Havana. The passengers were mainly

holiday-makers, from the cheaper end of the market according to the travel writer with whom I found myself seated. He, of course, was travelling free as the guest of the Cuban government, which was attempting to remedy a chronic shortage of Western currency by carving out for itself a niche in the Caribbean holiday trade. Tourism, they had discovered, was compatible with socialism after all.

We off-loaded the sun-seekers and scuba-divers, along with the travel writer, at Varadero. The few remaining passengers were mainly Cubans, privileged travellers who were coming home with half a department store of loot among them. Otherwise, there was only a Canadian couple, frowsily middle-aged, but purposeful in their way. Had they been to Cuba before? Indeed they had. Often. They translated in a voluntary capacity for the Ministry of Information in Havana. It was their contribution to the Revolution.

'How interesting,' I observed, unsure why they unnerved me. 'What kind of things do you translate?'

The woman pursed her lips as though she were guarding a state secret. But the man was more forthcoming. Actually, he said, they had just completed a small book dealing with the threat of AIDS, for distribution in the Anglophone countries of Africa. This puzzled me. What did the Cubans know about AIDS, or *el SIDA*, as he preferred to call it? It was true, he agreed, that the Cubans had only a limited experience of the disease. However, in contrast to the West, they had developed an energetic and progressive policy for dealing with it. The protection of public health was the number one priority. AIDS cases in Cuba were interned. Homosexuals. Soldiers. It made no difference.

'Interned?'

'Yes,' said the woman, her zeal for the Revolution still burningly intact. 'Interned. It is the most humane policy.'

I felt sick in the stomach.

At Havana I made arrangements to travel on without delay. I would go direct to Santiago, to Santiago where the poet Lorca heard the palms sing in the wind. From Santiago de Cuba the road runs east along the central valley of the province. The earth is red there, and over the emerald hills there rises a darker canopy of royal palms.

AFTERWORD

Within less than a year of the first publication of *Take Me to Paris, Johnny* in 1993, John Foster had died. Writing the memoir had consumed much of his time and energy in the years after Juan's death on Good Friday, 1987. He had earlier declined to have the AIDS test, not wishing to burden Juan with any pointless sense of guilt should the test have proved positive. Indeed, when, later, he did take the test, he still nursed a small hope that he might escape that diagnosis. It was not to be. At a time when the drug treatment of AIDS was still in its infancy, the immediate outlook for him was at best uncertain, and the need to tell the story of Juan became his primary concern. 'I have accomplished nothing,' was Juan's desolate reflection on his own life. For John it was important to 'accomplish' the book, as if to prove Juan wrong. It was necessary to go back to the beginning of it all, to make the trip to Cuba to meet Juan's mother, in preparation for which he learnt some Spanish. As he relates in the book, he came bearing a copy of my *Australia: A Cultural History*, a symbolic gesture because of its dedication to 'To John and Juan'.

Writing was never easy for John – yet he wrote so well

– and when he was struggling with the first draft he was greatly concerned that his family and straight friends might be offended, perhaps even shocked, by its depiction of gay life. There was the further problem that in writing about Juan he could not help also writing about himself, and he was not, by nature, given to self-disclosure. Having read the first draft, the publisher encouraged him to put more of himself into the text. John made a few conciliatory amendments but held back from revealing much more of his own story. In the end the publisher agreed that he had achieved the right balance.

And yet a careful reading of *Take Me To Paris, Johnny* tells us much about John Foster, his personality and pre-occupations. Its very tone – the subtle balance of formality and intimacy, of rationality and passion – conveys a real sense of the man, the historian, the teacher, the friend, the lover.

John had a secure, suburban childhood, but it was one he reacted against in adult life. Close as he was to his mother, he did not have happy memories of the family household. There was an atmosphere of penny pinching – understandable perhaps in a family of five children, with John the second eldest – and he would recall with a shudder the pudding-basin haircuts his father imposed on the three boys. He looked back at the family home as being culturally deprived: his father never read a book, took the *Sun*, and had few interests. It was a scholarship that took John from Elwood Park Central School to Wesley College. He had been baptised an Anglican, but had been sent to a Presbyterian Sunday school because it was closer, a common enough example of the Australian habit of regarding religion as a social convenience. At Wesley a friend (now an Anglican bishop) introduced him to Anglo-Catholic liturgy and worship, to which he was immediately attracted. However, at school and Melbourne University he was also a committed member of the inter-denominational Student Christian Movement. After gaining a Ph.D. in England, he returned to a History lectureship at Melbourne University, while for a few years also living in a monastic community associated with St Mark's, Fitzroy. The break with his suburban childhood could hardly have been more complete.

The brief dalliance with monasticism might, in the 1970s, have already marked him as an eccentric, but his return to the world did not signal a retreat from religion. As a student he had attended St Mary's Anglican Church, North Melbourne, and in 1978 he rented a house (and later a flat) which was part of the parish property. He became much involved in the affairs of the parish, particularly the beautifying of its Eucharistic worship which the recently inducted Father Jim Brady was developing, and John personally gave to the church candelabra, vestments, altar frontals, sanctuary lamps, a paschal candle stand (in memory of Juan) and much else. The importance for him of religion, and its expression through worship, permeates *Take Me to Paris, Johnny*, particularly noticeable in the way Juan's dying is contained within the narrative of Holy Week.

With religion went history. John's Ph.D. at the University of Wales, Swansea, was on the Anglican preacher and social reformer Canon Henry Scott Holland, but it was German history that was to become the main focus of his research and teaching, in particular the experience of German Jews and the trauma of the Holocaust and its legacy. As a small child he had been fascinated by some neighbours, a couple who were German Jewish refugees and who took an interest in him: their flat was decidedly exotic, filled as it was with strange furniture, rugs, china crockery, records and books, a foreign oasis in the suburban desert. In 1986, just a year before Juan's death, he was to edit an oral history collection, *Community of Fate: Memoirs of German Jews in Melbourne,* in which his childhood neighbours featured. His colleague and friend, the historian Mark Baker, has seen John's passionate interest in the Jews as reflecting his embrace of marginality, but it was also for him a creative dialogue between Christianity and its source in Judaism. On his death a rosary and a Jewish skullcap were found, side by side, in a drawer.

He was, by all accounts, a remarkable teacher. There was always the personal charm, of course, though he studiously avoided addressing undergraduates by their Christian names, preferring the respectful if slightly tongue-in-cheek formality of 'Mr' and 'Miss'. But there was also a sense of drama, an eloquence, and a total engagement with the historical reality with which he confronted students. In teaching a course on the Jewish Holocaust he did not forget its other victims, the gypsies, the Jehovah's Witnesses – and the homosexuals who, with little sense of group identity, were particularly vulnerable to the Nazis' persecution.

John's homosexuality was, however, basic to his own identity. I don't think that, given his religious temperament, he found it altogether easy to accept his sexuality, but he did, and he was honest and, at times, uncompromising about it. Many aspects of his personality make more sense, or perhaps a different kind of sense, when seen through the filter of his sexuality: his humour – and humours; his taste for the exotic; the interplay of strength and gentleness; his sense of mischief; his love of ritual. The ultimate expression of his sexuality was, of course, *Take Me to Paris, Johnny,* though it was not written for that purpose. But in telling the story of Juan, and of how the casual pick-up seamlessly became the affair and the lifelong commitment, he was also reflecting on his own needs, sexual and emotional.

Yet he was not by nature a gay activist. It was a little surprising, therefore, to find him turning up at a meeting in 1979 of the Gay Union of Tertiary Staff (GUTS proved, as it turned out, an inappropriate acronym), a Sydney-based organization which was attempting to set up a Melbourne branch. I had heard about John Foster but not met him before, and indeed I had got the impression that he was rather anti-social – and here was this charming, engaging, youngish man, a bit of a spunk in fact, with his neat, trim body, flashing smile, blue eyes and mop of blond hair. GUTS did not flourish, though for a time John had twinges of guilt that we were not doing more to sustain it. He was partly deterred by the ideological trappings the gay movement was acquiring, for which he had limited sympathy. Later, he did for a time convene a gay history seminar group, but there he was on comfortable home ground. And he enjoyed cultural expressions of gay life, whether in New York, Berlin or Melbourne, relishing the polarities of earnestness and out-rageousness, of innocence and sophistication.

Part of John's reputation as an eccentric stemmed from his Luddite tendencies. As far as much modern technology was concerned he was a conscientious objector. He would have no truck with computers, and in the library depended on the kindness of librarians to track down books. He didn't even countenance the typewriter, writing always in neat, understated longhand. As for ATMs, he detested their mechanical impersonality and would have nothing to do with plastic cards and pin numbers. He had once driven a car, but after an accident – which he (jokingly?) attributed to experiencing a vision of the Virgin Mary while at the wheel – gladly gave up on it. And in his pocket of North Melbourne, motor vehicles were definitely the enemy. When relieved of his watch in a poofter-bashing attack in a nearby park he did not bother to replace it, finding happily that he could rely on town hall clocks, church bells and the like. Perhaps his one concession to the technology of communications was his embrace of the telephone – he enjoyed the chat and gossip it facilitated.

Linked to his aversion to technology was his deep distrust of bureaucracy. This comes through strongly in *Take Me to Paris, Johnny* in the portrayal of Juan as a stateless person, treated with blank-faced indifference if not suspicion by immigration officials around the world. Mark Baker attributes John's hatred for bureaucracy to its association with the Holocaust; and technology could so easily be deployed as a means of state control. John resented any process that required the filling in of forms. He went for years without submitting a tax return, indifferent to the refunds that were probably owing to him. In the University he obstinately would not apply for the promotion to which he was surely entitled. And, according to fellow historian Greg Dening, 'he used not meeting deadlines as a sort of anti-bureaucratic espionage.'

John's lifestyle always retained a whiff of the monastic denial of money and possessions. As Jim Brady has observed, 'he liked to see a degree of extravagance and richness around him but not as part of himself.' John himself confesses in the memoir that money was a subject he had always found 'profoundly tedious'. As a tenured lecturer he always seemed to have enough: what he had he spent or gave away, 'a mildly profligate reaction against the thrift of a middle-class upbringing'. For Juan, who was always struggling to survive at the edge of New York's underclass, this was, as John wryly observed, irresponsible carelessness.

This kind of other-worldliness should not be taken to imply a lack of interest in his material surroundings. As a child he had a passion for plants, flowers, gardens. Granted early on his own vegetable and flower patch, he was soon taking much of the responsibility for the family's garden, stoutly defending it against his father's tendency to cut down anything showing signs of healthy life. Garden history became an important minor research interest and he gained a particular reputation as an authority on Melbourne's parks and gardens. In 1989 he published an edited collection of documents, *Victorian Picturesque: The Colonial Gardens of William Sangster*; as he mentions in the memoir, Juan helped him with some of the research. John was a popular speaker with the Garden History Society which he supported. And in the Australian suburban tradition, there was always room in John's garden for chooks; he even went so far as to join the Essendon Poultry Society.

He was not, however, an enthusiast for native plants, at least not in the urban environment. Street planting of untidy eucalypts, with their peeling bark and scraggy foliage, caused him great distress, and, indeed, brought out the urban terrorist in him, as he did not shrink from rooting them out under cover of darkness. In the garden, as in other areas of his life, he nursed his prejudices carefully. Describing the flowers brought by a friend to Juan in hospital, he applauds the bright colours of gerberas in spite of their emanating from racist South Africa, but compensates by declaring anathema 'the whole hideous tribe of the proteas'.

His engagement with parks and gardens was one aspect of his strong sense of place. He related very much to the local world of North Melbourne – the splendid, noisy profusion of the Victoria Market, the almost country-town atmosphere of Errol Street, the Italian exuberance of the neighbourhood trattoria, and, before it folded, the down-at-heel gay bar with its cheerfully amateur drag show. Melbourne University, within easy walking distance, also meant a lot to him. It had been the focus for his working life, and its nooks and crannies were as important to him as the collegial sociability it offered. Although he was occasionally lured to Monash to give a lecture, he greeted that car-infested suburban campus with a shudder. The bulk of his estate went to Melbourne University – to buy more books for the Library in his chosen fields.

Melbourne, in the larger sense, was also important to him. He was comfortable with the Melbourne brand of tribalism and was a strong supporter of the Collingwood Magpies, once confessing to me that it was the 'thuggish' players he was most drawn to. Melbourne, and, at a pinch, Victoria, had meaning for him: on the other hand he had a profound distaste for nationalism. Sydney was definitely foreign territory and he viewed its culture with suspicion. Looking abroad, he had a British disdain for things Irish, although one of his closest friends had an Irish background; and in North America he could feel entirely at home in New York while preferring not to see it as part of the United States. He loved Berlin, too, as is evident in *Take Me to Paris, Johnny*, and was able to detach his affection for the city, and particular parts of it at that, from any thought of German nationalism, which would have instantly conjured up the horrors of the Third Reich and the Holocaust. Always it was the immediacy of place and the people contained within it that evoked a response from him.

He was, then, a man of contradictions, many of which, I am sure, he was conscious of. Sometimes one wondered how serious his prejudices were; or at least it could be hard to distinguish those which were deeply felt from those which were adopted more playfully. He relished conversation but there was often an element of polite mischief in his contribution to it: he enjoyed the effect created by saying something slightly outrageous or politically incorrect and yet would profess mild astonishment at the reaction it elicited. Yet he could also be tactful in accommodating and adjusting to the views of others. Although not initially an enthusiast for the ordination of women he respected its importance for many of his friends and accepted its inevitability.

One had a feeling that the charm, the playfulness, the eloquence, masked a very private angst or self-doubt, something which he had sought to assuage in the monastic community and which was difficult to communicate to others. Like most of us, he had secrets, the most trivial one being that he smoked. His friends were not supposed to know: if caught with a cigarette in his hand the incident would not be referred to, and the fiction that he was a non-smoker maintained. He also reserved to himself the right to go his own way. He had no qualms about leaving a dinner party abruptly if he was tired of it, and more generally his comings and goings could be unpredictable, not helped, perhaps, by the lack of a watch. Eccentricity, one suspected, could be a refuge.

There was no disguising, however, the central integrity of his life. One reason why writing could be agonising for him was that he had such high expectations of it. I think, in this respect, writing the story of Juan offered a kind of release.

The emotion which underpinned it and the urgency of the project were sufficient to reassure him that the words on the page conveyed a truth that justified the act of writing. There was a sense, then, in which *Take Me to Paris, Johnny* was not only his tribute to his lover but Juan's final gift to him.

The launch of *Take Me to Paris, Johnny* on 2 September 1993 was a happy occasion. It was held at the Meat Market and a great crowd of John's family, friends and colleagues attended, all of whom sensed, I think, the importance of the moment. Dipesh Chakrabarty, then a member of Melbourne's History Department, spoke eloquently in launching the book, concluding by singing a song about love and grief by Tagore, the first song his mother had taught him. John responded with his usual grace and charm. He made a reference to a recent bout of sickness, and said that he had been overwhelmed by the support of friends. He felt he could face the future with confidence. It might have been an emotional moment for many in the audience, but John was adept at striking a note which overcame that danger.

Three weeks later John was hospitalised with a brain infection, toxo-plasmosis. When he emerged from a coma he was for a time disoriented, convinced at first that he was in Israel, then a Paris monastery, though you couldn't be quite sure that this wasn't a game he was playing with us. Although he made a partial recovery, he was never quite his old self again – yet what, one could not help wondering, was that old self? Certainly, aspects of the John we knew were recognisable through the haze of illness – as when, one evening, he arose from his bed in the Royal Melbourne Hospital and quietly walked out, and, somehow negotiating the hectic traffic of Flemington Road in pyjamas and Sandy

Stone dressing gown, headed home to Howard Street, where he was greeted with considerable surprise by friends enjoying a pre-dinner drink in the vicarage garden. For John it was as though he was simply making a sociable call and he offered no explanation for his unexpected arrival; he stayed for dinner, and, after an anxious phone call from the hospital to report that he had gone missing, made no objection when it was suggested that it was time for him to return.

Whereas Juan, the dancer, had, in his dying, seen his body wasting away to a skeleton, for John, the historian, there was the sad irony that his mind bore the brunt of AIDS. Adding to the tragedy, Murray, the vital young friend referred to in the book – it is Murray who brings Juan gerberas – was also hospitalised with AIDS-related illnesses at this time. John attended Murray's funeral just a month before his own death.

It all came to an end at St Mary's which, like the University, had been such an essential part of his life. There was the full requiem mass with all the ritual he would have wanted, though his body was contained in a simple Jewish-style coffin of unadorned pinewood. After the eulogies had been said, the hymns sung and the Eucharist celebrated, his body was borne to Kew Cemetery to join Juan. There, as had happened with Juan's burial, those gathered joined in filling in the grave. Remembering that earlier occasion, Greg Dening remarked that not many of us will turn the soil of their own grave as John did.

Yet, whatever one's beliefs, it was not the end. *Take Me to Paris, Johnny* survives as more than just a superbly crafted memoir – it is also a living expression of the spirit of John Foster.

It was Greg Dening who offered the beautiful prayer:

'Thank you, Lord, for John. May the gardens grow, the bantams hatch and the bell toll as John would have liked.'

John Rickard

Sources
Mark Baker's comments come from his Introduction to *History on the Edge: Essays in Memory of John Foster (1944–1994)*, History Department, University of Melbourne, 1997, which also contains funeral eulogies by Jim Brady and myself. Greg Dening is quoted from his speech launching *History on the Edge*, to be found in a booklet published by Saint Mary's Anglican Church in 1997, with the support of the Department of History, Melbourne University, entitled *Bell and Book: In Memoriam John Harvey Foster*. I am also indebted to Ross Foster for his recollections.